Functional Assessment of Urinary Neuro-biogenic Amines

A COMPREHENSIVE GUIDE

Andrea Gruszecki, ND

Table of Contents

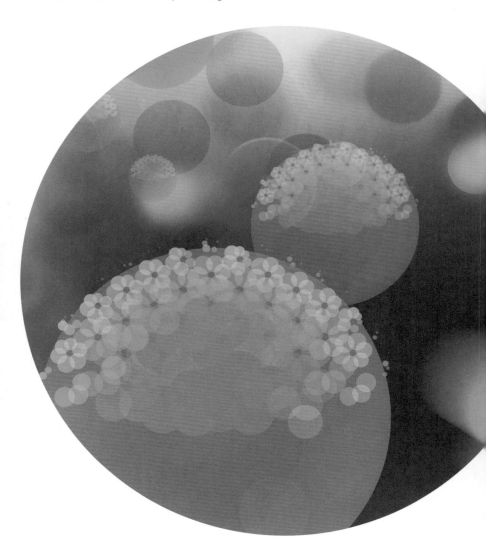

Functional Assessment of Urinary Neuro-biogenic Amines: A Comprehensive Guide

Doctor's Data, Inc. is pleased to offer Urinary Neuro-biogenic Amines testing. Urinary neuro-biogenic amines (neurotransmitters) are a non-invasive way to assess the status of neurotransmitter molecules essential for normal function. Information gained through neuro-biogenic amine testing may provide therapeutic opportunities that improve clinical success and patient health outcomes. Associations between urinary neurotransmitter levels and health conditions have been documented in scientific literature and may provide valuable insights as part of a comprehensive health assessment.

Urinary neuro-biogenic amines may serve as biomarkers for neurotransmitter status. Biomarkers [such as cholesterol, thyroid stimulating hormone (TSH) or complete blood count (CBC)] are commonly used in medical evaluations. Such measurements indicate biologic function, and may be used in both in patient assessment and to monitor the results of therapy. Complex disorders, such as diabetes, are often evaluated and monitored with just a few biomarkers. Urinary neurotransmitter biomarkers may provide additional insights for pa-

tients with behavioral, cognitive or neurologic symptoms. Altered patterns of urinary neurotransmitters may highlight the need for precursor amino acids or nutritional cofactors essential for synthesis and metabolism.

What is a Neuro-biogenic Amine (neurotransmitter)?

A neuro-biogenic amine is a molecule (chemical) that carries a signal between nerve cells. A neuromodulator is a molecule that alters a nerve cell's response to a *neurotransmitter* signal. Neuro-biogenic amines and neuromodulators have effect when they bind to specialized receptors on other cells, or inside a cell. Neurotransmitters are necessary because all nerve cells are separated by minute spaces called *synapses*. (See Figure 1.)

Neuro-biogenic amines convert the electrical signal that travels within the nerve cell into a chemical signal that is shared with another nerve cell. The receiving, or *post-synaptic* cell, then generates the electric signal to pass onto the next cell. The electrical signals, or *action potentials*, are generated in the nerve

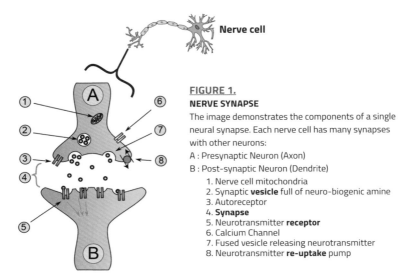

Nerve cell

<u>FIGURE 1.</u>
NERVE SYNAPSE
The image demonstrates the components of a single neural synapse. Each nerve cell has many synapses with other neurons:
A : Presynaptic Neuron (Axon)
B : Post-synaptic Neuron (Dendrite)
1. Nerve cell mitochondria
2. Synaptic **vesicle** full of neuro-biogenic amine
3. Autoreceptor
4. **Synapse**
5. Neurotransmitter **receptor**
6. Calcium Channel
7. Fused vesicle releasing neurotransmitter
8. Neurotransmitter **re-uptake** pump

Images courtesy of Wikimedia Commons. Synapse drawn by fr:Utilisateur:Dake with Inkscape 0.42. Used with permission.

cells by the passage of charged mineral elements, or ions, into and out of the cell. A lack of mineral elements may affect the function of nerve cells, and prevent proper electrical signaling.

In general, a neurotransmitter is synthesized by the nerve cell, then, stored in a *vesicle* until it is needed. There is always a small amount of neuro-biogenic amines leaking out of vesicles into the synapses; in a healthy nervous system this neurotransmitter released is either taken back into the nerve cell and vesicle or metabolized by enzymes in the synapse or nerve cell. Some nerve cell metabolites may act like neurobiogenic amines or neuromodulators. Other metabolites have no known function and are simply excreted from the body by the liver and kidneys. Normal levels of neurotransmitters are essential for nerve cell function in the central and peripheral nervous system.

The central nervous system (CNS) consists of the brain and spinal cord (Figure 2). The peripheral nervous system consists of all the nerve fibers that branch off from the spinal cord and extend to all parts of the body. The CNS is separated from the peripheral nervous system by the blood-brain barrier (BBB), a single cell lining around the brain's blood vessels and capillaries (Figure 2). The semi-permeable membrane barrier limits blood circulation access to the brain and spinal cord. The BBB is meant to protect the brain from foreign substances and infectious agents, to maintain a constant supportive environment for the brain, and to keep out hormones and neurotransmitters released into circulation.

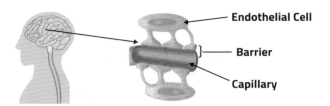

Endothelial Cell

Barrier

Capillary

FIGURE 2.

The central nervous system consists of the brain and spinal cord. The ***blood-brain barrier*** is a single layer of cells that protects the central nervous system from foreign substances in the circulating blood.

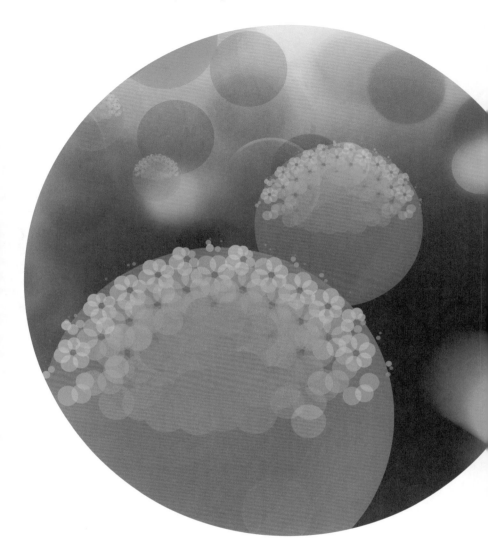

Types and Functions of Neuro-biogenic Amines

There are many types of neuro-active substances. "Classic" neurotransmitters are called small molecule neurotransmitters or biogenic amines. Some amino acids obtained from the diet or synthesized in the body may act as neurotransmitters or neuromodulators. Other amino acids serve as precursors for neurotransmitter synthesis. Many peptides (proteins formed by linked amino acids) are neuro-active, and many hormones have neuro-active properties. The neurotransmitters tested by Doctor's Data, Inc. include precursor and neuro-active amino acids, "classic" small molecule neurotransmitters and their metabolites:

- **Small molecule neurotransmitters (biogenic amines)**
  - Catecholamines: Dopamine, Epinephrine (Adrenalin), Norepinephrine
  - Histamine, Serotonin
- **Metabolites**
  - 3,4-Dihydroxyphenylacetic acid (DOPAC), 3-Methoxytyramine (3-MT), 5-Hydroxyindolacetic acid (5-HIAA), Metanephrine, Normetanephrine
  - Trace Amines: Phenylethylamine (PEA), Tyramine, Tryptamine

- **Amino acids**
  - Gamma aminobutyric acid (GABA), Glutamate, Glycine, Taurine, Tyrosine

Neurotransmitter function is determined by the molecule's post-synaptic effects. (See Figure 1.) Neurotransmitters act in two ways, they either increase (excitatory) or decrease (inhibitory) the likelihood that a nerve cell will transmit any electrical information. Multiple neurotransmitters may be released together into a single synapse. The neurotransmitters released together may serve as "co-transmitters". As co-transmitters they may further influence a nerve cell or receptor's response to neuro-active compounds. Excitatory neurotransmitter synapses have a different conformation (form) and location on the nerve cell from inhibitory synapses. Only two neurotransmitters, the amino acids GABA and glycine, have inhibitory effects. The levels of neurotransmitters are determined by their rates of synthesis and metabolism (breakdown), or turnover. The effect of a neurotransmitter is determined, in large part, by the receptor that it binds to.

Neurotransmitter Transporters

Monoamine transporters are located in cell membranes and include specific transporters for dopamine (DAT), norepinephrine (NET) and serotonin (SERT). The transporters move monoamines into and out of cells using ion gradients. The transporters function to remove neurotransmitters from the synapse ("reuptake") back into the cell for storage in vesicles. The neurotransmitters are removed from the cytoplasm into vesicles by the vesicular monoamine transporter (VMAT). Mutations and single nucleotide polymorphisms in monoamine transporters may affect neurotransmitter levels and are being evaluated for their effects in behavioral, mood, attention and neurodegenerative disorders. Inhibition of monoamine transporters by "reuptake inhibitor" medications is used in the treatment of depression, obsessive compulsive disorder (OCD), anxiety, chronic pain syndrome, and attention deficit hyperactivity disorder (ADHD). Altered VMAT density in the brain has been associated with neurodegenerative conditions.

Neurotransmitter Receptors

Neurotransmitter activity occurs when a neuro-active molecule binds to specific receptors on the post-synaptic nerve. (See Figures 1 & 3.) Receptor function is as important as neurotransmitter levels; a dysfunctional receptor may affect biochemistry, mood, behavior and learning. Receptors are specialized proteins on neurons. Two main types of receptors, excitatory and inhibitory, determine the response of a signal-receiving neuron. A balance between excitatory and inhibitory signaling is necessary for normal function. Excessive excitatory signaling may result in symptoms

such as seizures, excessive inhibitory signaling may result in sedation, anesthesia or loss of coordination.

The binding of a neurotransmitter to a receptor activates its function. Receptor activation may have direct effects on the nerve cell or activate second messengers. Second messengers may have local or systemic effects. The activity of a nerve cell is determined by the balance of excitatory and inhibitory signals it receives. Often, a neurotransmitter may have the ability to bind to several types of receptors. Some receptors are "promiscuous" and may bind with multiple neurotransmitters. Other compounds, such as hormones and drugs, may also bind to neurotransmitter receptors. At least one receptor type, the N-methyl-D-aspartate receptor (NMDAR), binds two neurotransmitters simultaneously. NMDA receptors bind to glutamate, but also require a glycine cofactor. (See Figure 3.)

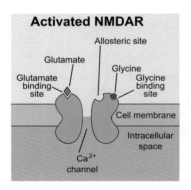

Image courtesy of Wikimedia Commons. Image by RicHard 59 with Inkscape. Used with permission.

FIGURE 3.

The binding of a neurotransmitter to its receptor activates a receptor function, in this example, opening an ion channel.

There are two primary types of neurotransmitter receptors, *ionotropic* and *metabotropic*. Ionotropic receptors open or close channels in the cell membrane to allow ions (such as calcium) to enter or leave the cell. Changing the level of ions in a cell affects the cell's potential to generate electrical signals (see Figure 3). Metabotropic receptors affect cell activity indirectly through second messengers. Second messengers may have local or systemic effects. Local second messenger effects might involve changes in nerve cell chemistry or DNA expression to make the cell more or less likely to transmit information. Second messenger pathways include the cyclic AMP (adenosine monophosphate) pathway, the inositol triphosphate/diacylglycerol (IP3/DAG) pathway and the arachidonic acid pathway.

The number, structure and function of neurotransmitter receptors may be affected by mutations or single nucleotide polymorphisms (SNPs), which may alter the amount of time a neurotransmitter stays bound, and the ease of binding. It is possible for neurotransmitter levels to be normal, and still have symptoms, if the receptor is dysfunctional. Neurotransmitter receptor defects have been associated with mood disorders, bipolar disorders, and addictive behaviors. Research continues to determine how receptor dysfunctions might contribute to neurodegenerative disorders such as Alzheimer's, Parkinson's and Huntington's disease.

Neuro-biogenic Amine Synthesis and Metabolism

Urinary neuro-biogenic amines provide an overall assessment of a patient's ability to synthesize and metabolize neurotransmitters, which must occur in both the peripheral nervous system and behind the blood brain barrier (BBB) in the central nervous system (CNS). Altered patterns of urinary neuro-biogenic amines may highlight the need for precursor amino acids or nutritional cofactors essential for synthesis and metabolism. The assimilation and absorption of nutrients requires a healthy digestive tract and a healthy microbiome (the presence of expected and beneficial microbes in the gastrointestinal tract). Neurotransmitters arise from amino acid precursors (see Figure 4.)

Some neuro-biogenic amine precursors are essential amino acids that must be obtained from the diet. Other neurotransmitters may be synthesized by the body, and are considered non-essential. The essential amino acid precursors are **phenylalanine** and **tryptophan**. Mutations or single nucleotide polymorphisms (SNPs) may alter enzyme conformation or function and affect the synthesis of neuro-biogenic amines. The enzymes in the synthesis pathway require nutrient cofactors; the nutrients will be reviewed in the specific information for each neurotransmitter. However, three important enzymes, phenylalanine hydroxylase (PAH), tyrosine hydroxylase (TH) and tryptophan hydroxylase (TPH) begin the synthesis process. All three enzymes require a tetrahydrobiopterin (BH4) cofactor, and all incorporate iron into their structures. Defects in BH4 synthesis or recycling may affect neurotransmitter synthesis and nitric oxide signaling. BH4 deficiency may present with elevated levels of precursor amino acids and low levels of neurotransmitters. Enzymatic defects in methylation capacity (methionine metabolism and transsulfuration pathways), may affect BH4 levels and may increase oxidative stress in the CNS. Oxidative stress may

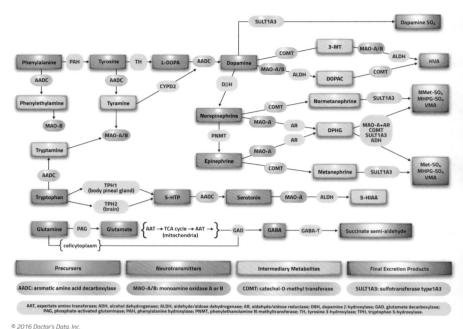

© 2016 Doctor's Data, Inc.

FIGURE 4.
Neuro-biogenic amine metabolism.
Metabolism of neurotransmitters inside nerve cells occurs primarily via a two-step process using MAO-A and various dehydrogenase and reductase enzymes. COMT is not found in sympathetic nerve cells.

also alter the level of neurotransmitters and enzyme functions.

The metabolism of catecholamine neuro-biogenic amines often takes place in the same cells where the amines are produced. This occurs because catecholamines are constantly leaking out of vesicles and then taken up again by the neurons. Circulating neurotransmitters may also be metabolized in the liver or kidney. The enzymes in the pathway often require nutrient cofactors; the nutrients will be reviewed with their neurotransmitters. The metabolism of precursors or neurotransmitters results in intermediary metabolites. The metabolites may or may not be biologically active, but may provide important functional clues

about certain enzymes, such as catechol-O-methyl transferase (COMT) or monoamine oxidase (MAO). Mutations or single nucleotide polymorphisms (SNPs) may alter enzyme conformation (shape) or function and affect the metabolism of neurotransmitters. Different enzymes may be used, and different metabolites generated, if a neurotransmitter is processed within a neuron (intraneuronal) or outside it (extraneuronal). (Figure 5.)

There are two forms of monoamine oxidase (MAO). Monoamine oxidase A (MAO-A) activity is necessary for **intra**neuronal neurotransmitter metabolism. It oxidizes the catecholamine neuro-biogenic amines dopamine, norepinephrine and tryptophan to an aldehyde intermediary. MAO-A also oxidizes dietary and environmental amines. Aromatic amines are common ingredients in dyes, pigments, insecticides and polymers. Dopamine is oxidized by MAO A and B. Increased MAO-B activity has been associated with aging and Parkinson's disease. MAO is inherited with the X chromosome; males have one copy and females have two copies of the genetic instructions for MAO. Inherited variations in MAO activity may affect neurotransmitters or neurochemistry. Various mutations and single nucleotide polymorphisms (SNPs) have been associated with autism, behavior, attention, mood and bipolar disorders. In addition to medications designed to inhibit MAO activity (MAOIs), MAO

may be inhibited by cigarette smoke. Animal studies indicate that MAO activity may upregulate with stress. Toxic elements, and excessive levels of essential elements, such as copper and iron, may also inhibit MAO function.

Catechol-O-methyltransferase (COMT) activity is necessary for extraneuronal neurotransmitter metabolism. COMT methylates both catecholamines and catecholamine metabolites oxidized by MAO. (See Figure 5.) High levels of COMT are found in the liver and kidneys; COMT is also found in red blood cells and in adrenomedullary chromaffin cells. Various mutations and SNPs in the genes coding for COMT have been associated with some types of mood disorders, obsessive-compulsive disorder and schizophrenia. Research

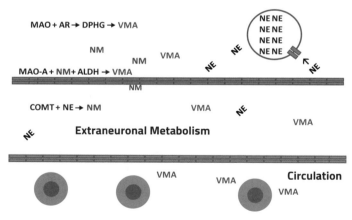

Image by Andrea Gruszecki ©2015 Doctor's Data, Inc.

FIGURE 5.
Monoamine oxidase A (MAO-A) is found inside sympathetic nerve cells. Catechol-O-methyltransferase (COMT) is not found in sympathetic nerve cells. A neuro-biogenic amine, norepinephrine (NE) in this example, is actively taken into vesicles within the nerve cell for storage, however, small amounts of neurotransmitter are constantly leaking out of the vesicles. NE metabolized by MAO-A will produce different metabolites than NE metabolized by COMT.

Legend: ALDH = aldehyde dehydrogensase; AR = aldose/aldehyde reductase; DPHG = 3,4 dihydroxyphenylglycol; NM=normetanephrine; VMA = vanilylmandelic acid.

continues to determine if other COMT SNPs may be associated with neurodegenerative disorders, cognitive disorders, or behavior disorders. COMT requires magnesium and S-adenosyl methionine (SAM) cofactors.

Intraneuronal metabolism occurs primarly via a two-step process through MAO-A and various dehyrodrogenase and reductase enzymes. Extraneuronal metabolism occurs through MAO, COMT and sulfotransferase (SULT) enzymes. COMT is not found in sympathetic nerves, but is abundant outside the neuron in other cells and tissues. Mutations or single nucleotide polymorphisms (SNPs) may occur in the dehydrogenase or reductase enzymes, and may affect enzyme function. Some of these secondary enzymes may produce neurologically active metabolites.

- Aldehyde dehydrogenase (ALDH) activity contributes to a variety of vital biochemical reactions in the body. Altered ALDH function is associated with a variety of medical conditions such as Sjogren's syndrome, type II hyperprolinemia, -hydroxybutyric aciduria, and pyridoxine-dependent seizures. ALDH is part of the metabolic pathway for dopamine and serotonin. Two dopamine metabolites may elevate and have neurotoxic effects due to increased oxidative stress if ALDH function is compromised. Deficient ALDH activity may contribute to elevations of 3-methoxytyramine and serotonin. Environmental aldehydes that must be processed by aldehyde dehydrogenases include cigarette smoke, formaldehyde, polyurethane, polyester plastics, and medications. Aldehyde excess due to enzymatic insufficiency may be associated with symptoms of dizziness, nausea, rapid heartbeat (tachycardia) and "alcohol flush".

- Alcohol dehydrogenase (ADH) converts alcohols into aldehydes or ketones that must then be metabolized by ALDH. ADH may participate in the conversion of Vitamin A into retinoic acid.

- Aldose reductase (AR)/Aldehyde reductase (ALR) – reduces aldehyde metabolites of neurotransmitters, aldehydes, corticosteroids, and xenobiotic aldehydes from environmental exposures. These enzymes are abundant in the liver and kidney.

Neuro-biogenic amine synthesis or metabolism may be altered by the presence of other medical conditions. Evaluation of these neurotransmitters should be considered for patients with a history of myocardial infarct (heart attack), diabetes, hypothyroid or adrenal disorders. Rarely, urinary neurotransmitters may confirm the presence of certain tumors. Neurotransmitter levels may also be influenced by diet, lifestyle and other factors such as high sodium intake, age, gender, body mass index, kidney function, detoxification capacity, environmental exposures, infection or tobacco use. Final excretion products are the result of liver or kidney detoxification. Urinary Neuro-biogenic Amine testing presumes normal kidney function; urine results may be compromised by kidney disorders.

Because metabolic enzymes are expressed differently in various body tissues, circulating levels of the biogenic amine neurotransmitters and their metabolites may have distinctive sources. For example, dopamine and norepinephrine metabolism occurs primarily in the gastrointestinal tract (GIT) Urinary levels of neurotransmitters pri-

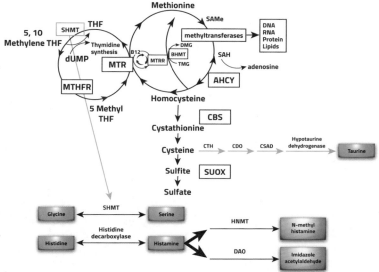

Image by Andrea Gruszecki © 2015 Doctor's Data, Inc.

FIGURE 6.

Synthesis of non-catecholamine neurotransmitters.

Synthesis of Glycine, Histamine and Taurine

The methylation pathway (as it is commonly known) synthesizes cysteine behind the blood-brain barrier, and is a precursor for the antioxidants taurine and glutathione.

Legend: AHCY = adenosylhomocysteinase; BHMT = betaine-homocysteine methyltransferase; CBS; CTH = cystathionine gamma lyase; CDO = cysteine dioxygnase; CSAD = cysteinesulfinic acid decarboxylase; DAO = diamine oxidase; HNMT = histamine N methyltransferase; MTR = methionine synthase; MTRR = methionine synthase reductase; MTHFR = methylenetetrahydrofolate reductase; SHMT = serine (glycine) hydroxymethyltransferase; SUOX.

marily reflect the activity of the peripheral and GIT enteric nervous systems. Up to 20% of some urinary neurotransmitters are estimated to originate in the CNS. However, as the enzymatic machinery for neurotransmitter synthesis and metabolism is often similar, if not identical, on both sides of the blood-brain barrier (BBB), normalizing urinary neurotransmitter levels based on test results has been shown to result in the improvement of some mood and behavior symptoms.

Not all neurotransmitters are synthesized through the same pathways. Glucose metabolism leads to the biosynthesis of neurotransmitters such as glutamate, and gamma-aminobutyric acid (GABA). Specialized support cells in the brain, the astroglia (astrocytes) contribute to the synthesis and metabolism of glutamate and GABA (see Figure 6).

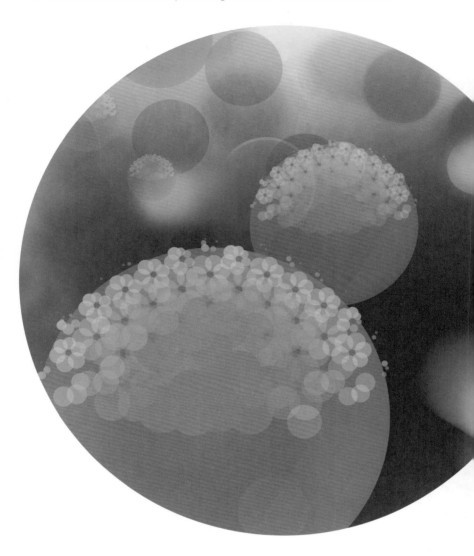

Blood-Brain Barrier

The blood-brain barrier (BBB) is a semi-permeable membrane that separates the central nervous system (CNS) from peripheral blood circulation. (See Figure 2.) Normal BBB function is necessary for normal brain function. The BBB functions to:

Protect the brain from foreign substances and infectious agents

Buffer fluctuations of neuro-active compounds, nutrients and elements in the systemic circulation to maintain a constant environment for the brain

Keep out hormones and neurotransmitters released into systemic circulation; excess that might over-stimulate brain receptors and disrupt central nervous system signaling

Regulate the migration of circulating immune cells into the brain

The BBB exists as tight junctions between specialized capillary endothelial cells that line the blood vessels and capillaries of the brain. Astroglia (astrocyte) cells surround the blood vessels. Astroglia also act as a partial barrier while providing nutrient support to the capillary endothelial cells and the nerve cells of the brain. The endothelial capillary wall further employs efflux pumps, which actively transport unwanted molecules back into blood circulation. In the CNS astroglia may release neuro-active molecules (cross-talk), supply neurons with neurotransmitter precursors, sequester or metabolize extracellular neurotransmitter molecules or respond to neurotransmitter signaling.

Water and lipid (fat)-soluble substances pass through the BBB easily, and a variety of transport mechanisms exist to ensure that the brain receives the nutrients it needs. Other transport mechanisms ensure that CNS wastes are released back into the circulation. Large molecules, polar (charged) molecules and charged ions cross the BBB with difficulty unless they are specially transported. In addition to the barrier and efflux pumps, enzymes found on the capillary endothelial cell walls further filter the substances passing into the brain. Mutations or single nucleotide polymorphisms may affect the structure or function of these enzymes or transport mechanisms.

There are several areas of the brain where the BBB is more permeable or absent. These areas, called cirumventricular organs, allow the brain to monitor the blood composition (feedback) to make adjustments to the body physiology. The BBB may be damaged, which increases its permeability and allows foreign substances into the brain. The presence of foreign substances from the circulation, such as bacterial lipopolysaccharides or environmental toxins, may cause inflammatory changes in the brain; these changes may affect mood and behavior. Accumulating evidence points to associations between BBB dysfunction and the progression of a variety of CNS diseases, such as stroke, multiple sclerosis, brain tumors or neurodegenerative diseases such as Parkinson's or Alzheimer's diseases. The BBB tight junctions may be damaged by:

- High blood pressure
- Delayed development (the BBB is not fully formed at birth)
- Radiation
- Infection
- Inflammation
- Trauma (injury)
- Oxidative stress
- Low oxygen (hypoxia)
- Post-hypoxia re-oxygenation

The enzymatic machinery for neurotransmitter synthesis and metabolism is often similar, if not identical, on both sides of the BBB, and normalizing neurotransmitters has been shown to result in the improvement of some mood and behavior symptoms. Because metabolic enzymes are expressed differently in various body tissues, circulating levels of neurotransmitters and their metabolites may have distinct sources. For example dopamine and serotonin synthesis and metabolism occurs primarily in the gastrointestinal tract (GIT). Glia cells are found in the enteric (gut) nervous system and in muscle tissue as well as in the CNS. Glial cells in the enteric nervous system may be part of the gut mucosa, may be associated with enteric ganglia (nerve cell clusters), or may be associated with enteric nerves in the smooth muscle layers of the gut. Urinary levels of neurotransmitters primarily reflect the activity of the peripheral and GIT enteric nervous systems. Up to 20% of urinary neurotransmitters are estimated to originate in the CNS.

Endogenous Effects

Lifestyle and environment may contribute to neurotransmitter function or imbalance. Altered patterns of urinary neurotransmitters may highlight the need for precursor amino acids or nutritional cofactors essential for synthesis and metabolism. The assimilation and absorption of nutrients requires a healthy digestive tract and a healthy microbiome (the presence of expected and beneficial microbes in the gastrointestinal tract). The metabolism of neurotransmitters requires functional detoxification pathways and metabolic enzymes. Neurotransmitter levels may be influenced by diet, medications, nutrition status, lifestyle and other factors such as high sodium intake, age, gender, body mass index, kidney function, detoxification capacity, environmental exposures, infection, tobacco use, stress and inheritance.

Diet

Foods and beverages may contain neuro-active molecules that may bind to neurotransmitter receptors and alter neurotransmitter levels or have other effects. Monosodium glutamate (MSG), a common food flavoring agent, is known to bind to glutamate receptors. Disorders of digestion and absorption may result in malnutrition; low levels of amino acid precursors and enzyme nutrient cofactors may affect neurotransmitter synthesis or metabolism. The gastrointestinal bacteria (microbiome) may also synthesize and metabolize neuro-active compounds. A healthy microbiome may contribute to neurotransmitter balance through gut-brain-microbiome communications. A diet full of nuts, seeds, legumes, fresh fruits and vegetables provides the fibers required by beneficial and expected flora. (See **Digestion and Absorption** section.)

Due to the industrialization and over-processing of food, the diet is now a potential avenue of exposure to monosodium glutamate (MSG), preservatives, artificial colors and flavors. Calorie-dense, nutritionally depleted foods are common fare, and diets rich in such processed foods have been associated with depression and behavior issues in some studies. Research continues in this area.

- Diets that eliminate allergens and intolerances (oligoantigenic or "elimination" diet) have been shown to decrease attention deficit hyperactivity disorder (ADHD) symptoms in multiple studies. One study from the Netherlands correlated the elimination diet, immunoglobulin G (IgG) food antigen tests and ADHD symptoms, with relapse of ADHD symptoms upon food challenge in 63% of children.

- Studies indicate that a subpopulation of children may be sensitive to artificial food dyes; symptoms of exposure may include irritability, sleep problems, inattention, impulsivity, and hyperactivity. The reactions may not be restricted to children with ADHD, but may occur in the general population. Three genes, histamine degradation gene polymorphisms HNMT T939C, HNMT Thr105Ile and dopamine transporter gene DAT1 polymorphism (short versus long) have been associated with susceptibility to food dyes. Blue #1 food dye is known to cross the blood brain barrier.

- Ketogenic diets are high in fat and low in carbohydrates; this diet is used to minimize symptoms and seizures in epileptic patients. Studies indicate that some ADHD children have epileptiform brainwave discharges. Animal studies indicate that ketogenic diets may decrease activity levels.

Diets rich in fruits, vegetables, and healthy fats that avoid highly processed foods, food allergies or intolerances, and that employ more traditional cooking methods (such as steaming) have been consistently associated with improved health and decreased risk of chronic, degenerative diseases.

Certain foods should be avoided for at least three days prior to neurotransmitter testing. Different foods may contain neuro-active compounds or affect

the synthesis or metabolism of different neurotransmitters. In addition, patients should avoid cold weather conditions before and during testing and ensure proper hydration with water or fluids. Catecholamine (dopamine, epinephrine, norepinephrine) levels may be affected by:

- Alcohol
- Amines
  - Walnuts, avocados, fava beans, cheese, beer, red wine
- Banana
- Chocolate
- Citrus fruits
- Cocoa
- Coffee
- Cola
- Licorice
- Tea
- Vanilla
Serotonin levels may be affected by:
- Avocado
- Bananas
- Eggplant
- Fruit (especially those listed)
- Kiwi fruit
- Nuts (especially those listed)
- Pineapple
- Plums and prunes
- Tomato products
- Walnuts

Medication

Medications may alter neurotransmitter levels by binding to or blocking neurotransmitter receptors. **No medication should ever be discontinued without the permission of the prescribing physician.** Sudden discontinuation of certain medications may be hazardous to health.

Neuro-active medications are designed to alter neurotransmission; used according to prescription and under medical supervision, such drugs may provide relief for a variety of behavioral, mood and psychiatric disorders. These drugs may act by:

- Altering the rate of neurotransmitter clearance from the synapse

- Altering the rate of release of neurotransmitter from a neuron

- Binding with a receptor the same as a neurotransmitter

- Blocking a neurotransmitter from binding with a receptor

- Alter the flow of ions (minerals) into and out of neurons

- Inhibiting synthetic enzymes

Most medications are intended to affect a certain neurotransmitter pathway or receptor, however, other pathways and receptors may be inadvertently affected. In addition, no neurotransmitter signaling system exists in isolation; a specific neurotransmitter or receptor may send and receive signals that affect other neurotransmitter pathways. Additional side effects may occur if neuro-active medications are taken inappropriately or in conjunction with other neuro-active compounds such as herbs or vitamins.

Environmental exposure may occur when neuro-active compounds are found in discharge from water treatment plants. A recent study found evidence of antivirals, antibiotics, muscle relaxants, antidepressants, tranquilizers, medications for treating cancer, diabetes, and hypertension in ground water below a waste treatment plant. Another study found neuro-active compounds, such as antidepressants, anti-seizure compounds, and mood stabilizers in 24 rivers across Minnesota.

Medications designed for other uses may sometimes have neurological side effects:

- Antihistamine medications alter the levels of histamine, an important neurotransmitter in the brain, causing drowsiness.

- Antibiotics may have neurotoxic side effects, and present with a wide variety of neurological symptoms. Individuals of advanced age and those with kidney insufficiency, liver disease or prior central nervous system disease may be most vulnerable to such side effects.

- Steroids, produced by the body or taken as medication, may affect neurotransmitter receptors and influence the release of glutamate, gamma-aminobutyric acid (GABA), acetylcholine, norepinephrine, dopamine and serotonin.

Drugs of abuse disrupt neurotransmission. While many drugs disrupt particular neurotransmitters or pathways, most drugs of abuse directly or indirectly enhance dopamine signaling in reward pathways. An excellent overview of the effect of drugs of abuse on neurotransmission may be found on the National Institute on Drug Abuse website: *http://www.drugabuse.gov/news-events/nida-notes/2007/10/impacts-drugs-neurotransmission*

Medications that may alter catecholamine (dopamine, epinephrine, norepinephrine) testing include:

- acetaminophen (Tylenol®)
- aminophylline
- amphetamines
- appetite suppressants
- caffeine
- chloral hydrate
- clonidine

- dexamethasone
- diuretics
- epinephrine
- insulin
- imipramine
- lithium
- methyldopa
- monoamine oxidase (MAO) inhibitors
- nicotine
- nitroglycerine
- decongestant nose drops
- propafenone
- reserpine
- salicylates (aspirin)
- theophylline
- tetracycline
- tricyclic antidepressants
- vasodilators

Medications that may alter serotonin levels include:

- morphine
- monoamine oxidase (MAO) inhibitors
- reserpine
- methyldopa
- lithium
- serotonin re-uptake inhibitors
- tryptophan or 5-hydroxy tryptophan (5-HTP) supplements

No medication should ever be discontinued without the permission of the prescribing physician. Sudden discontinuation of certain medications may be hazardous to health.

Digestion and Absorption

The gastrointestinal tract (GIT) has its own nervous system. The enteric (GIT) nervous system is sometimes call a "second brain"; fibers from the GIT travel directly to the central nervous system via the vagus nerve. Ninety percent of the fibers in the vagus nerve originate in the gut and travel to the brain. The vagus nerve is part of the autonomic ("visceral") nervous system. The autonomic nervous system regulates involuntary activity such as digestion, blood pressure and respiration. Disorders may originate in the autonomic nervous system or result from another disease such as diabetes or Parkinson's disease. Altered neurotransmitter levels may contribute to autonomic enteric nervous system disorders in the GIT. In addition to GIT-specific neuro-active compounds, the gastrointestinal tract responds to signals from catecholamines (dopamine, epinephrine, norepinephrine), serotonin and melatonin. Mood disorders may alter the levels of gastrointestinal hormones, such as somatostatin and vasoactive intestinal peptide (VIP). Alterations in GIT hormone signaling may contribute to irritable bowel syndrome (IBS). Peripheral dopamine and norepinephrine metabolism occurs primarily in the gut. Sulfotransferase (SULT) 1A3 is one of three metabolic pathways for dopamine, and is found in the gastrointestinal tract and colon. (See Figure 4.)

Urinary levels of neurotransmitters primarily reflect the activity of the peripheral and GIT enteric nervous systems. Digestion, motility, immunity, permeability and absorption of nutrients may affect neurotransmitter synthesis, or be affected by, alterations in neurotransmitter levels or disorders of the autonomic nervous system.

The gastrointestinal bacteria (microbiome) is known to synthesize and metabolize both neuro-active compounds and essential vitamins (biotin, Vitamin K, etc.). A healthy microbiome may contribute to neurotransmitter balance through gut-brain-microbiome communications. A diet full of fresh fruits, vegetables, nuts, seeds, and legumes provides the fibers required by beneficial and expected flora. The microbiome may be disrupted by alterations in neurotransmitters or GIT functions. Germ-free mice are often used in GIT-microbiome studies. Germ-free mice are raised in sterile conditions and have sterile guts; there are no gastrointestinal bacteria present in these animals. Studies comparing germ-free mice and mice with pathogen-free microbiomes indicate that a normal microbiome directly affects the levels of free catecholamines (dopamine, epinephrine, norepinephrine) in the gut.

The presence of pathogens or dysbiotic species in the microbiome may disrupt normal gut functions and increase intestinal permeability. Some species of *Clostridia* bacteria *(C. bolteae, C. histolyticum, C. limosum, C. bifermentans, C. novyi A, C. sordelli, C. subterminae)* have been associated with neurological and developmental disorders. The toxic metabolites may escape into the circulation and cross the blood-brain barrier (BBB), where they may disrupt normal neurological functions. If intestinal permeability is increased, the likelihood of toxic metabolites, bacterial lipopolysaccharides (cell wall proteins) and large dietary proteins escaping into the systemic circulation increases. If the blood-brain barrier is also compromised, then central nervous system (CNS) inflammation may result. Loss of normal intestinal permeability has been associated with gastrointestinal and systemic inflammatory conditions. Inflammatory changes in the CNS have been associated with increased CNS oxidative stress and changes in mood and behavior. CNS inflammation may also downregulate cytochrome P450 enzyme functions. Digestion, motility, the microbiology of the gut and the integrity of the intestinal barrier may be evaluated by laboratory testing. More information about these tests is available at *www.doctorsdata.com.*

Comprehensive Stool Analysis w/Parasitology x3

Intestinal Permeability

Comprehensive Clostridium Culture

Evaluation of the gastrointestinal microbiome should be considered an essential part of any patient evaluation for mood, behavior or psychiatric disorders. Animal studies have clearly demonstrated the effects of acute and chronic stress on the gastrointestinal system. Stress or disrupted neurotransmitter signaling in the gut may induce changes in immune functions, inflammatory pathways and microbiome populations. Expected and beneficial bacteria work together in species groups or "guilds". Species within microbiome guilds provide a common enzymatic function for the gastrointestinal system. A loss of diversity (loss of populations) of expected and beneficial species groups may disrupt:

- digestion and absorption
- synthesis or metabolism of neuro-active compounds
  - altered levels of neuro-active compounds may disregulate gut-brain-microbiome communication
- microbial methylation and detoxification
- production of nutritive short chain fatty acids for the gut cells
- normal gut-microbe interactions
- tolerance (normal anti-inflammatory and immune system functions)
- intestinal permeability

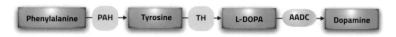

FIGURE 7.
Phenylalanine is converted to tyrosine by the enzyme phenylalanine hydroxylase (PAH).

The correction of digestive disorders and microbiome insufficiency may be necessary to ensure the absorption and assimilation of nutrient cofactors that may be used to correct neurotransmitter disorders. Digestive health may be evaluated through laboratory testing. More information about these tests is available at *www.doctorsdata.com.*

Comprehensive Stool Analysis w/Parasitology x3

Intestinal Permeability

Microbiology Profile

Renal Function and Neurotransmitters

The precursor amino acid phenylalanine is converted to tyrosine by the enzyme phenylalanine hydroxylase (PAH). The kidney is the primary source of circulating tyrosine; approximately 50% of phenylalanine conversion (for the whole body) occurs in the kidneys (see Figure 7). Kidney disease may affect the levels of neurotransmitters in urine. A Creatinine Clearance test may be done to evaluate kidney function prior to other urine tests. More information about this test is available at *www.doctorsdata.com.*

Creatinine Clearance

Endocrine and Metabolic Effects on Neurotransmission

Endocrine hormones affect the function of neurons in the central nervous system (CNS), and may influence neurotransmission. Changes in the hypothalamus-pituitary-adrenal axis may alter neurotransmission, hormone levels and physiology, as may thyroid and sex hormones.

Parathyroid disorders disrupt calcium metabolism. Mild hypercalcemia may contribute to depression, apathy, irritability and lack of spontaneity. Severe hypercalcemia may result in symptoms of psychosis, lethargy or catatonia, and may progress to coma. Mild hypocalcemia may contribute to symptoms of anxiety, parasthesias, irritability and emotional lability. Severe hypocalcemia may result in symptoms of mania, psychosis, and seizures.

Thyroid disorders may be associated with changes in mental status. Depression is a common symptom in hypothyroid (low) conditions, and anxiety may be seen in hyperthyroid (high) conditions. Thyroid supplementation is a common treatment for mood disorders. Hypothyroid conditions have been shown to decrease responses to serotonin and decreased serotonin 5-HT2A receptor density and sensitivity. Thyroid hormone levels may be evaluated in the laboratory. More information about this test is available at *www.doctorsdata.com.*

Thyroid Profile

The association of metabolic dysregulation and neuropsychiatric symptoms has been demonstrated in both human and animal studies. Normal insulin levels are necessary for neuron growth, health, plasticity and regulation. "Sugar reactions" in children may be a symptom of reactive hypoglycemia, which may impair cognitive function and attention. Such reactions may be mitigated by including a quality protein source for all meals and snacks.

Metabolic disturbances, such as insulin resistance, diabetes and obesity are associated with neurodegenerative disorders. Alterations in neuron function may be due to abnormal insulin signaling in the central nervous system (CNS), and may contribute to diseases such as Alzheimer's. Psychiatric disturbances and metabolic dysregulation are commonly associated, and may be found together in depression, schizophrenia, and neurodegenerative disorders such as dementia, Alzheimer's, Parkinson's and Huntington's disease. Congenital neurodegenerative and neurological disorders may also have concurrent metabolic dysregulation. Long term corticosterone (glucocorticoid) exposure decreases insulin sensitivity in animal models. Glucorticoids may be produced by the body during stress (cortisol) or introduced into the body as medication (cortisone, hydrocortisone). Chronic high levels of glucocorticoids may disregulate insulin responses and blood sugar, which predisposes for insulin resistance (metabolic syndrome) and type II diabetes. Animal studies demonstrate that glucocorticoid administration induces insulin resistance and depressive behavior. Stress-related insulin dysregulation and depression are associated with increased risk of Alzheimer's disease. Levels of insulin, and other biomarkers of metabolic dysregulation, may be assessed in the laboratory. More information about this test is available at *www.doctorsdata.com*.

Metabolomic profile

Adrenal disorders may contribute to neurological, mood or psychiatric symptoms. Cushing's Syndrome (adrenal over-function) may result in symptoms of depression, anxiety, mania, psychosis, or cognitive dysfunction. Neuropsychiatric symptoms may present before physical symptoms. Addison's Syndrome (adrenal under-function) may result in symptoms of apathy, lack of pleasure (anhedonia), fatigue and depression. Adrenal insufficiency may be mistaken for major depressive disorder.

Maternal lead exposure, or exposure to lead during development, may permanently alter the hypothalamus-pituitary-adrenal axis (HPA), which controls stress responses. Exposure to toxic elements may be evaluated in the laboratory. More information about these tests is available at *www.doctorsdata.com*.

Urine Toxic Elements

Whole Blood Elements

Hair Toxic and Essential Elements

Dysregulation of sex hormones other hormones may affect moods and neurotransmission.

- Growth hormone, in excess may result in symptoms of mood lability, depression and personality changes.

- Prolactin, in excess, may depress libido and contribute to feelings of depression or anxiety.

- Testosterone, if deficient, may decrease libido in both genders and contribute to depression in women.

- Estrogen directly influences brain function; estrogen receptors are located on neurons in multiple areas of the brain. Estrogen increases the concentration of catecholamine neurotransmitters (dopamine, epinephrine, norepinephrine) and modulates the rate of neurotransmitter turnover. Estrogen also seems to promote the expression of neurotransmitter receptors. Estrogen inhibits monoamine oxidase (MAO). Estrogen is considered anti-inflammatory, which may protect the brain. Estrogen levels are associated with changes in mood and behavior in women. Particularly after menopause, low estrogen levels have been associated with increased depression.

- Progesterone has multiple functions in the central nervous system; it regulates cognition, mood, mitochondrial function, neurogenesis and neuro-regeneration. These functions are mediated by progesterone receptors found in the brain and on all neural cell types.

Nutrient Cofactors

Nutrient status, from diet or supplements, may affect neurotransmitter synthesis and metabolism, and thereby, nervous system functions. Studies indicate a correlation between increased mental health disorders and the adoption of a Western diet (high in saturated fats, red meat, and simple carbohydrates). Western diets tend to be higher in processed "empty-calorie" foods and low in fruits, vegetables and fiber. Deficiencies in essential nutrients have been associated with mood, behavior

and psychiatric disorders. Nutrient status may also affect medication dosing. Research is ongoing to determine how nutrient therapies may affect biochemistry, physiology, mood, behavior and cognitive functions. At least one study has correlated improved nutrient status with better Global Assessment of Functioning (GAF) scores in patients diagnosed with psychiatric disorders.

A review by Booij, Van der Does, and Riedel (2003) on the effects of acute (short-term) amino acid precursor depletion in healthy and psychiatric populations indicates that there may be specific effects based upon which precursor amino acids are depleted in the volunteer's plasma. The effects of amino acid depletion were modified by both the length of time in symptom remission and the presence or absence of psychiatric medications, such as selective serotonin reuptake inhibitors (SSRIs), etc. Not all patient populations were studied with every type of amino acid depletion. Very few placebo effects were reported from the control populations. The review reported that in multiple studies:

- The effects of amino acid depletions – tryptophan, tyrosine or phenylalanine/tyrosine – were neurochemically specific and affected specific neurotransmitter systems rather than general brain metabolism

- Tryptophan depletion
  - tended to lower mood in depressed patients being treated with SSRI medications and in patients considered recovered
  - diminished memory executive functions in psychiatric patients but not in healthy controls
  - decreased REM sleep and melatonin secretion

- Both tryptophan and tyrosine depletion lowered mood in Seasonal Affective Disorder (SAD) patients
- Tyrosine depletion
  - increased positive (psychotic) symptoms in schizophrenia patients
  - impaired attention
- Phenylalanine/tyrosine depletion impaired memory

The effects described in the review consider only the effect of precursor amino acid depletion. The synthesis and metabolism of neurotransmitters involves a variety of enzymes, many of which require specific nutritional cofactors. The chart below provides a brief review of some of the nutrients that may affect neurotransmitter synthesis, metabolism or function. Studies indicate that many patients with mood or psychiatric disorders use non-prescription nutritional supplements in attempts to improve health or minimize side effects. The results of one study found that 66% of study participants were using at least one non-prescription product, and 58% were taking non-prescription nutritional supplements in combination with neuro-active medications. Such combinations may result in adverse effects unless prescribed and supervised by a medical professional.

Nutritional status may be assessed by laboratory testing. More information about these tests is available at *www.doctorsdata.com.*

Urine or Plasma Amino Acids

Red Blood Cell (RBC) Elements

Urine Iodine

Whole Blood Chromium & Vanadium

The following supplements may be used by clinicians to support patients with neurological, behavioral or mood symptoms or patients with imbalanced neurotransmitters. Supplements should only be used with the consent and supervision of a clinician to avoid adverse reactions or effects.

- **Consult with your physician and pharmacist to avoid any potential adverse effects or drug/nutrient interactions prior to starting or stopping any nutrient or drug therapy.**

- **No medication should ever be discontinued without the permission of the prescribing physician. Sudden discontinuation of certain medications may be hazardous to health.**

- **The chart is not intended to diagnose or recommend any specific nutrient as a treatment.**

NUTRIENT	AFFECTS	EFFECTS	CONCERNS	AVAILABLE TESTS
Fatty Acids Ω-3 Ω-6			Doses higher than 3 gm daily may affect clotting times and increase bleeding risks. **May interact with medications and other health conditions.**	
Essential fatty acids	Neuron cell membranes Hormone Second messengers	Required for normal vision and neural development. Dietary deficiencies during gestation and development may result in pathology or functional deficits; essential for normal cognition. Ω-3 fatty acids have been shown to reduce plasma catecholamine levels. May improve symptoms of psychiatric, neurological and neurodegenerative disorders.	Doses higher than 3 gm daily may affect clotting times and increase bleeding risks. May interact with medications.	**Fatty Acids; Erythrocytes**
a-linolenic acid Ω-3	Second messengers Synapse membranes	DHA precursor; deficiency is associated with defects in CNS function, visual system; Ω-3 fatty acids may have antidepressant effects. Ω-3 deficiency has been associated with post-partum depression.	Contraindicated in personal or family history of prostate cancer. May increase high trigylcerides. No established daily upper limit.	**Fatty Acids; Erythrocytes**

NUTRIENT	AFFECTS	EFFECTS	CONCERNS	AVAILABLE TESTS
DHA Ω-3 Docosahex-aenoic acid	Second messengers Synapse membranes	Deficiency has been associated with defects in CNS function, visual system; human studies demonstrate improvements with depressive, bipolar, schizophrenia symptoms when given with EPA. Ω-3 deficiency has been associated with post-partum depression.	DHA may counteract beneficial EPA effects in schizophrenia. May affect blood sugar levels. No established daily upper limit.	Fatty Acids; Erythrocytes
EPA Ω-3 Eicosapen-tanoic acid	Second messengers Synapse membranes	Deficiency has been associated with defects in CNS function; human studies demonstrate improvements with depressive, bipolar, schizophrenia symptoms when given with DHA. Ω-3 deficiency has been associated with post-partum depression.	Doses higher than 3 gm daily may affect clotting times and increase bleeding risks. May be contraindicated with aspirin therapy. May interact with antihypertensives.	Fatty Acids; Erythrocytes

NUTRIENT	AFFECTS	EFFECTS	CONCERNS	AVAILABLE TESTS
Vitamins			Doses of fatty Vitamins A,D,E and K that exceed daily upper intake limits may have adverse health effects. **May interact with medications and other health conditions.**	
Biotin	Enzyme cofactor	Deficiency has been associated with depression, fatigue, hallucination, parasthesia (tingling in extremities).	Inherited disorder may affect holocarboxylase synthetase and ability to use biotin. Anti-seizure medications, antibiotics, may decrease biotin levels. Digestive disorders may decrease biotin levels. No established daily upper limit.	
Choline or Phosphatidyl choline	Acetylcholine	Precursor compound for acetylcholine. Deficiencies have been associated with tardive dyskinesia and similar movement disorders; may be used in neurodegenerative and psychiatric disorders.	Exceeding tolerable upper intake limit (3.5 gms daily for adults) may result in adverse health effects.	

NUTRIENT	AFFECTS	EFFECTS	CONCERNS	AVAILABLE TESTS
Folates/ folic acid	Cell metabolism, enzymes and methylation	Deficiency has been associated with depression. Methylation defects are associated with altered neurotransmitter metabolism, mood & psychiatric disorders, autism, neurodegenerative diseases, neural tube defects, increased oxidative stress. Some methylation defects may contribute to tetrahydrobiopterin deficiencies.	Exceeding tolerable upper intake limit (adults 1,000 mcg daily) may result in adverse health effects and neurologic symptoms.	**Methylation Profile; plasma**
(alpha) Glycerophos-phocholine	Cell membranes	Evidence indicates mild improvements in cognitive functions in early Alzheimers, dementia, and vascular brain injury.	Average dose for human studies is 400mg three times daily. No tolerable upper limit established.	
Tetrahydrobi-opterin (BH4)	Redox status/ oxidative stress. Enzymes and methylation.	Cofactor for neurotransmitter synthesis and metabolism enzymes. BH4 deficiencies have been associated with increased oxidative stress, neurodegenerative diseases, and in some phenylketonuria patients.	Administration affects nitric oxide (NO) synthesis and may affect heart and vascular signaling and function. Upregulates hydroxylase enzymes for Phenylalanine, Tyrosine and Tryptophan. No established upper limit for oral administration. Supplements may not cross the BBB.	

NUTRIENT	AFFECTS	EFFECTS	CONCERNS	AVAILABLE TESTS
Vitamin A	Vision Retinoid signaling	Deficiency has been associated with anxiety and depression. Animal studies indicate Vitamin A needed for normal neural development.	Toxic if tolerable upper limit (adult 10,000 IU daily) exceeded. Contraindicated with liver disease and Type V hyperlipoproteinemia.	
Vitamin B-1 (thiamine)	Cell metabolism, enzymes	Deficiency has been associated with axon degeneration, cardiovascular symptoms, peripheral neuropathy, pain in lower extremities and back progresses to sensory loss and loss of reflexes and motor control. Deficiency has been associated with mood disorders in women. Deficiency has been associated with cognitive decline in elderly.	No established upper limit for oral administration.	
Vitamin B-2 riboflavin	Cell metabolism, enzymes and methylation.	Deficiency has been associated with depression.	No established upper limit for oral administration.	**Methylation Profile; plasma**
Vitamin B-3 niacin	Cell metabolism, enzymes and methylation Redox status/ oxidative stress	Deficiency has been associated with dementia, increased oxidative stress. Neuroprotective. Animal studies indicate that B-3 may attenuate the progression of neurodegenerative diseases.	Liver damage has been reported with unsupervised high doses or timed-release formulations. Exceeding the tolerable upper daily limit (adults 35mg/day) may cause adverse health effects. Large doses of nicotinamide may cause methyl donor depletion.	**Methylation Profile; plasma**

NUTRIENT	AFFECTS	EFFECTS	CONCERNS	AVAILABLE TESTS
Vitamin B-6 (pyridoxal -5-phosphate or P5P)	Cell metabolism, enzymes and methylation Aromatic amino acid decarboxylase (AADC)	Deficiency has been associated with depression.	Exceeding tolerable upper limit (adults 100 mg daily) may have adverse health effects and result in sensory neuropathy.	**Methylation Profile; plasma**
Vitamin B-12	Cell metabolism, enzymes and methylation	Deficiency has been associated with dementia, loss of language and cognitive functions. Deficiency has been associated with peripheral neuropathy, loss of motor control, increased reflexes.	Therapy must begin prior to symptoms to delay cognitive decline and dementia. No established upper limit for oral administration.	**Methylation Profile; plasma**
Vitamin C	Redox status/ oxidative stress DβH enzyme	Antioxidant. Vitamin C deficiency has been associated with bipolar disorders to protect against excess Vanadium. Used to treat Tyrosinemia.	High oral doses may result in diarrhea. High doses are contraindicated in certain health conditions, including iron overload disorders.	**DNA Oxidative Damage Assay**
Vitamin D	Serotonin synthesis General metabolism Gene expression Immune functions	Deficiency has been associated with incidence of multiple sclerosis (MS); mood and cognition in elderly; depression, psychiatric disorders and dementia.	Exceeding tolerable upper intake limit (adult 4,000 IU daily) may have adverse health effects. Medications may affect Vit. D metabolism or absorption.	**Vitamin D serum** **Vitamin D bloodspot**
Vitamin E	Redox status/ oxidative stress	Deficiencies associated with reflex abnormalities, sensory neuropathy, peripheral neuropathy, radiculopathy.	Exceeding tolerable upper intake limit (adult 1,500 IU) may affect clotting times and increase bleeding risks.	**DNA Oxidative Damage Assay**

NUTRIENT	AFFECTS	EFFECTS	CONCERNS	AVAILABLE TESTS
Amino Acids			**Excessive levels of amino acids may cause brain damage and intellectual disability.** **May interact with medications and other health conditions.** No established upper limits; all available through diet.	
GABA	GABA receptors	Direct supplementation to correct deficiency.	May be contraindicated with neuro-active or antidepressant medications.	
Lysine	Enzyme function	Deficiency may prevent use of Vitamin B-6 by cells.	Excess may inhibit arginase and nitric oxide signaling.	**Plasma Amino Acids** **Urine Amino Acids**
Phenylalanine	Catecholamines (Dopamine, Epinephrine, Norepinephrine)	Precursor amino acid for Tyrosine and Phenylethylamine (PEA).	Contraindicated in phenylketoneuria (PKU); excess may contribute to brain damage and intellectual disabilities.	**Plasma Amino Acids** **Urine Amino Acids**
SAMe (S-adenosyl-methionine)	Cell metabolism, enzymes and methylation	Methylation defects are associated with altered neuro-transmitter metabolism, mood & psychiatric disorders, autism, neurodegenerative diseases, neural tube defects, increased oxidative stress. Some methylation defects may contribute to tetrahydrobiopterin deficiencies.	SAMe supplementation may alter liver detoxification and affect the half-life, effects and dosage requirements of medications. May be contraindicated with certain methylation enzyme defects.	**Methylation Profile; plasma**

NUTRIENT	AFFECTS	EFFECTS	CONCERNS	AVAILABLE TESTS
Taurine	Neurons/receptors	Neuromodulator — regulates flow of ions into and out of nerve cells. Deficiency associated with bipolar disorders; may counter effects of excess acetylcholine.	Excess or deficiency may damage heart, kidney, liver, pancreas, retina. Taurine supplements may alter kidney function (like a diuretic) and affect lithium levels in those using prescription lithium.	**Plasma Amino Acids** **Urine Amino Acids**
Tyrosine	Catecholamines (Dopamine, Epinephrine, Norepinephrine)	Precursor amino acid for catecholamine and Tyramine synthesis. Converts into thyroid hormone.	Tyrosine may be contraindicated in thyroid conditions.	**Plasma Amino Acids** **Urine Amino Acids**
Tryptophan	Serotonin	Precursor amino acid for Serotonin and Tryptamine synthesis.	Uses same transport mechanism into brain as other precursor amino acids. Give separately on empty stomach or with carbohydrates to maximize absorption.	**Plasma Amino Acids** **Urine Amino Acids**

NUTRIENT	AFFECTS	EFFECTS	CONCERNS	AVAILABLE TESTS
Minerals			Excess or deficiency of mineral cofactors may have adverse effects. **May interact with medications or other health conditions.**	
Calcium	Action potential (nerve firing) Electrolyte balance	Studies indicate supplements may improve moods in premenstrual syndrome.	Exceeding tolerable upper intake limit (adult 2,000 mg daily) may have adverse health effects. Serotonin re-uptake inhibitor (SSRI) anti-depresssant medications may inhibit bones from absorbing Calcium. Serum Calcium levels may be increased by Lithium therapy and may have adverse health effects.	**Red Blood Cell (RBC) Elements** **Serum Elements**
Chromium (Cr3+)	Blood sugar regulation	Deficiencies have been associated with depression and poor control of carbohydrate cravings.	Deficiency may be misdiagnosed as mood disorder. No established tolerable upper limit established; high levels may have adverse health effects.	**Whole Blood Chromium & Vanadium**
Copper	Enzyme function DβH enzyme	Deficiency has been associated with muscle weakness, peripheral neuropathy, loss of motor control, increased reflexes, optic neuropathy, loss of myelin sheath in CNS. Excess may increase oxidative stress in the brain.	Contraindicated in Copper-storage diseases. Exceeding tolerable upper intake limit of 10mg daily (adults) may have adverse health effects and has been shown to damage kidneys.	**Red Blood Cell (RBC) Elements**

NUTRIENT	AFFECTS	EFFECTS	CONCERNS	AVAILABLE TESTS
Iodine	Thyroid function	Deficiency may contribute to hypothyroid disorders.	Exceeding tolerable upper limit (adults 1.1 mg daily) may have adverse effects on thyroid function. Hypothyroid symptoms may be misdiagnosed as mood disorder.	**Urine Iodine** **Urine Halides**
Iron	Red blood cells, enzymes	Cofactor for enzymes, anemia has been associated with bipolar disorders, restless leg syndrome and febrile seizures. Excess may increase oxidative stress in brain.	Exceeding tolerable upper limit (adults 45 mg daily) may result in iron overload. Iron overload may damage heart, liver, kidney, pancreas and result in neurogenerative conditions. May be contraindicated in Iron-storage disorders, thalessemias, sickle cell disorders.	**Red Blood Cell (RBC) Elements** **Serum Elements**
Lithium	Serotonin	Interacts with physiology and biochemistry. Moderates neuron excitability. May have neuro-protective effects. Used to treat mood and psychiatric disorders; may alter Serotonin levels.	Doses exceeding 100 mg daily (adults) have been associated with adverse health effects. No established tolerable upper limit. May cross-react with medications. May be contraindicated by heart disease, kidney disease, thyroid disease. Contraindicated in pregnancy and nursing. Blood levels need to be monitored.	**Whole Blood Elements**

NUTRIENT	AFFECTS	EFFECTS	CONCERNS	AVAILABLE TESTS
Magnesium	Enzymes	Cofactor for many essential synthesis and metabolism enzymes	Exceeding tolerable upper limit intake (adults 350 mg daily) may have adverse health effects. Oral doses may result in diarrhea or gastrointestinal symptoms.	**Red Blood Cell (RBC) Elements**
Molybdenum	Enzymes	Incorporated into Iron or pterin-containing cofactor complexes required by multiple enzyme groups. Mutations in molybdenum cofactor protein have been associated with neurological symptoms.	Exceeding the tolerable upper limit (adult 2 mg daily) may have adverse health effects. Synthesis of molybdenum enzyme cofactor requires s-adenosyl-methionine (SAM) and normal methylation pathways. High doses have induced Copper deficiency in animals.	**Red Blood Cell (RBC) Elements** **Methylation Profile; plasma**
Selenium	Enzymes	Deficiency has been associated with anxiety, depression. Deficiency increases risk of age-related cognitive impairment.	Toxic if tolerable upper intake limit (adults 400mcg daily) is exceeded or used long-term.	**Red Blood Cell (RBC) Elements**
Zinc	Enzymes	Deficiency has been associated with poor cognition, depression, Alzheimer's and psychiatric disorders in older patients. Required for mental and motor development in children.	May potentiate anti-depressant medications. Exceeding tolerable upper intake limit (adults 40mg daily) may interfere with copper absorption and have adverse health effects. Neuroprotective properties lost if Zinc in excess.	**Red Blood Cell (RBC) Elements**

NUTRIENT	AFFECTS	EFFECTS	CONCERNS	AVAILABLE TESTS
Herbs & Plant-based nutrients			**May interact with medications and other health conditions.** Safety and efficacy of most herbal products during pregnancy or breast-feeding has not been established.	
Forskolin *Coleus forskohlii*	Cell membrane ion channels (action potentials)	Animal studies indicate anticonvulsant effects for some chemically induced seizures. Increases levels of neurotrophin-3, which supports neuron growth and survival.	No established dose or tolerable upper intake limit established. May lower blood pressure and increase bleeding risks.	**DNA Oxidative Damage Assay**
Curcumin *Curcuma longa*	Redox status/ oxidative stress	Improved redox status (decreased oxidative stress); animal and in vitro studies indicate: 1) use in neurodegenerative diseases 2) may decrease proliferation of brain tumor cells.	No established dose or tolerable upper intake limit established. Oral doses poorly absorbed. Doses exceeding 8000 mg/day not well tolerated in studies. Effective dose/ administration routes not currently established in scientific literature.	**DNA Oxidative Damage Assay**
Flavonoids and plant polyphenols	Redox status/ oxidative stress SULT1A3 Cell signaling	Anti-oxidant and anti-depressive effects in animal studies. May downregulate SULT1A3 enzyme expression.	No established dose or tolerable upper intake limit established. Obtain from fruits and vegetables in diet.	**DNA Oxidative Damage Assay**

NUTRIENT	AFFECTS	EFFECTS	CONCERNS	AVAILABLE TESTS
Ginkgo biloba	Circulation	Increases blood flow to the brain. Early research indicates Gingko may improve symptoms of dementia, generalized anxiety disorder (GAD), and schizophrenia (in combination with mediction). May improve cognitive function in multiple sclerosis. Limited evidence for autism, ADHD, migraine.	Monitor blood pressure, blood sugar. May increase the risk of bleeding. May alter half-life of mediciations. May be contraindicated if using antidepressant medications or St John's wort. No established dose or tolerable upper intake limit established.	
L-theanine (green tea leaves)	Neuroprotective Memory & learning Moderates stress responses (human study)	May increase levels of serotonin, dopamine, GABA. May block or downregulate glutamate receptors. (animal studies)	May decrease blood pressure and exacerbate effects of antihypertensive medication. May decrease the effect of stimulant medications.	
Mucuna puriens	Dopamine receptors	Human study found seed powder similar in effect to L-DOPA medications.	May interfere with conventional medications in a similar manner to L-DOPA medications. May interfere with conventional Parkinson's treatments.	
Passion flower *Passiflora incarnata*	Neurotransmitter receptors	Animal studies indicate anti-anxiety effects. In vitro studies indicate binding of GABA receptors.	Contraindicated if sedative medications are used. May potentiate the action of MAO inhibitors (MAOI). May increase the risk of bleeding. No established dose or tolerable upper intake limit established.	

NUTRIENT	AFFECTS	EFFECTS	CONCERNS	AVAILABLE TESTS
Pycnogenol (pine bark extract)	Catecholamines (Dopamine, Epinephrine, Norepinephrine) Glutathione Immune response	Improved redox status (decreased oxidative stress); has been shown to normalize some catecholamine levels in ADHD; improved glutathione ratios.	May increase the risk of bleeding. May alter blood sugar regulation. No established dose or tolerable upper intake limit established.	**DNA Oxidative Damage Assay** **Glutathione; erythrocytes**
Rhodiola rosea	Redox status/ oxidative stress Neurotoxicity	Animal studies indicate Rhodiola may have anti-inflammatory effects; may attenuate effects of L-glutamate –induced neurotoxicity.	No established dose or tolerable upper intake limit established.	**DNA Oxidative Damage Assay**
St John's wort *Hypericum perforatum*	Serotonin or Serotonin receptors	May be as effective as serotonin-reuptake inhibitor medications for mild-moderate depression.	Large doses may cause sun photo-sensitivity. Contraindicated during pregnancy and breastfeeding. May interact with or affect repro-ductive hormones; may contribute to infertility. May interact with ADHD medications methylphenidate. Possible contribu-tion to symptoms of mania in psychi-atric disorders. In combination with serotonin reuptake inhibitor (SSRI) anti-depressants may cause Sero-tonin Syndrome. No established dose or tolerable upper intake limit established.	

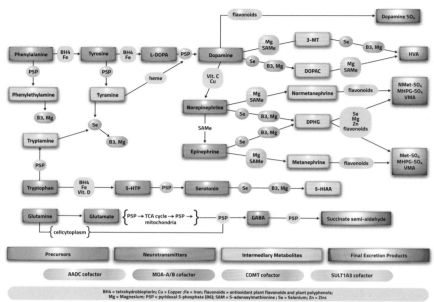

© 2016 Doctor's Data, Inc.

FIGURE 8.

Neurotransmitter Synthesis Nutrient Cofactors; Catecholamines and Serotonin

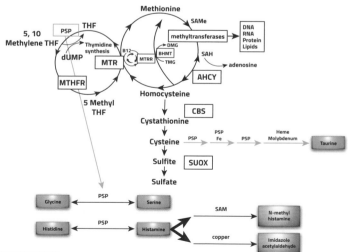

Image by Andrea Gruszecki © 2015 Doctor's Data, Inc.

FIGURE 9.

Synthesis of Glycine, Histamine and Taurine Nutritional cofactors.

The methylation pathway (as it is commonly known) synthesizes cysteine behind the blood-brain barrier, and is a precursor for the antioxidants taurine and glutathione.

Legend: AHCY = adenosylhomocysteinase; BHMT = betaine-homocysteine methyltransferase; CBS; Fe = iron; MTR = methionine synthase; MTRR = methionine synthase reductase; MTHFR = methylenetetrahydrofolate reductase; P5P = vitamin B6; SAM = S adenosylmethionine; SUOX

Environment, Exposures, and Inheritance

Inheritance and Epigenetics

An individual's inheritance the sum of the genetic material received from both parents. Genetic information controls the assembly and function of:

- Enzymes that synthesize neurotransmitters

- Enzymes that metabolize (degrade) neurotransmitters

- Transporters that move neurotransmitters, amino acids and nutrient cofactors across the blood brain barrier (BBB), into vesicles for storage, or across cell membranes

- Neurotransmitter receptors

The structure of deoxyribonucleic acid (DNA) may be altered by rare mutations. Mutations occur when an error is made by a cell during the copying of DNA (see Figure 10) the error may be due to:

- Alteration of a single base pair in the DNA

- Deletion of a base pair or larger section of DNA

- Insertion of extra base pairs into DNA

- Rearrangement of sections of DNA or chromosomes

Mutations are extremely rare. Another type of genetic variation, single nucleotide polymorphism (SNP), is much more common. SNPs are present in at least one percent of the popula-

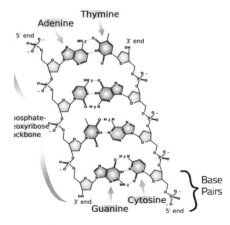

Image courtesy of Wikimedia commons.
Created by User:Madprime (2007) Used with permission.

FIGURE 10.
The structure of deoxyribonucleic acid (DNA); mutations occur when an error is made by a cell during the copying of DNA.

tion; some SNPs are far more common. Certain SNPs may affect the function of enzymes in biochemical pathways, others do not affect physiology or biochemical functions. Enzyme functions can often be improved if necessary nutritional cofactors are present; in a well-nutritioned individual, the effect of a SNP may be negligible. Not all functional SNPs affect enzymes, however, SNPS may affect neurotransmitter transporters or receptors as well.

The interaction of inheritance and the environment is termed *epigenetics*. The effects of diet, nutrition, toxic exposures and stress may all alter the expression of genetic information without re-writing the genetic code. Some examples of epigenetic environmental exposures include birth complications, maternal malnutrition, winter births, birth and growth in a large city, poverty, or relationships with family members (high-risk children). Some epigenetic exposures may occur pre-birth such as a maternal influenza infection during pregnancy, or drinking alcohol during pregnancy. Many types of epigenetic exposures have been associated with changes in behavior and neurologic processes in animal studies. Research continues in this area.

DNA expression is modified by the addition of molecules or "tags", such as S-adenosylmethionine (SAM) to DNA. Epigenetic changes occur when chemical modifiers, such as methyl or acetyl groups, are attached to DNA or to the structures that read, maintain and repair DNA. There is some evidence that an epigenetic alteration may be passed to offspring if the epigenetic effect induces a mutation is in a germline cell (sperm or egg), or if certain epigenetic tags are not erased during embryo development.

The epigenome allows an organism to respond to environmental changes through adaptation and evolution, as gene expression is upregulated or downregulated by intra- and extra-cellular signaling. A variety of cellular signals may induce epigenetic changes:

- Cytokines – the level and type of cytokines produced by the body determine the level of inflammation in a body tissue, organ or system

- Growth factors – proteins that stimulate cell growth, proliferation, repair and differentiation

- Hormones – such as cortisol, are known to alter gene expression; hormones may regulate the expression of epigenome-modifying genes

- Stress-response factors – protein complexes that repress the expression of genes activated by altered growth conditions or cellular stress

- Neurotrophic factors – such as brain-derived neurotrophic factor (BNDF), are proteins that support the growth and survival of mature neurons

Epigenetic changes may also occur due to malnutrition, over-nutrition or environmental exposures.

There are known associations between certain epigenetic DNA modifications and neurologic disorders in both developing and mature brains. Evidence indicates that epigenetic modifications in the adult brain may affect learning and memory-controlled behaviors, as well as synapse plasticity (capacity for new learning). Research indicates that epigenetic modification may not be static in the brain, but may change in response to changing conditions or neuron activation. Epigenetic modifications have been associated with neurodegenerative diseases such as Alzheimer's disease and Huntington's disease. Research indicates that epigenetic modification may also contribute to psychiatric disorders, mood disorders and additive behaviors.

One type of epigenetic DNA modification, methylation, attaches a methyl group to the DNA strand. The methyl group acts as an off switch, and prevents the expression of the gene until it (the methyl group) has been removed. If there are too few methyl groups are attached to DNA, then the mutation rate of the DNA may increase. An increased mutation rate has been associated with increased cancer risk. If too many methyl groups are attached to the DNA, then the organism may lose the response flexibility it needs to adapt to changing environmental conditions.

Methylation

The primary methyl group donor molecule in the body is S-adenosylmethionine (SAM). SAM is produced during the metabolism (breakdown) of the essential amino acid methionine (see Figure 11). Homocysteine, the product of the methionine metabolic pathway, is a necessary precursor for another essential amino acid, cysteine, which is synthesized in the trans-sulfuration cycle. Glutathione (GSH) is the primary antioxidant synthesized in the body; it is synthesized from cysteine, glycine and glutamate. Cysteine may also be converted into taurine, another amino acid essential for normal central nervous system (CNS) function. The synthesis of cysteine behind the blood brain barrier (BBB), and its conversion

to GSH, is essential to prevent oxidative stress and damage to the CNS.

SAM is the methyl donor in many transmethylation reactions in the body, including hormones, neurotransmitters, DNA, RNA, and phospholipids. SAM is the methyl donor used by the methyltransferase enzymes that synthesize neurotransmitters (such as norepinephrine, epinephrine, dopamine, serotonin, and histamine). Normal SAM levels may be required for the maintenance of myelin (the fatty layer of insulation that surrounds each nerve). Studies have shown that SAMe supplements may help reverse demyelination. Studies also indicate that SAMe oral supplements may be effective in the treatment of depression. Animal studies have demonstrated increased levels of norepinephrine and serotonin in the brains of rats given SAMe. SAM levels may also improve cell membrane fluidity and some membrane receptor functions. Other lines of research implicate SAM deficiency as contributing to the development of Alzheimer's disease.

The enzymes of methionine metabolism and the trans-sulfuration pathway (commonly termed the "methylation pathway") are prone to inherited genetic variation. Single nucleotide polymorphisms (SNPs) in the genetic code for methylation pathway enzymes may alter the enzyme's structure and function. Many of the enzymes on the methylation pathway require nutritional cofactors, such as B vitamins or minerals. The methylation pathway is important behind the blood brain barrier (BBB) to provide cysteine, taurine and GSH to neurons and glial cells.

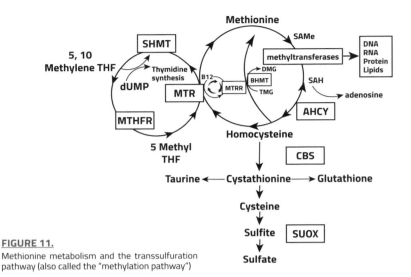

FIGURE 11.
Methionine metabolism and the transsulfuration pathway (also called the "methylation pathway")

While there is currently no method to evaluate or control the attachment of methyl groups to DNA, evaluation of oxidative stress and the methylation pathway (genetics and function) is available through laboratory testing. More information about these tests is available at *www.doctorsdata.com*.

DNA Methylation Pathway

DNA Oxidative Damage Assay

Methylation Profile; plasma

Glutathione; erythrocytes

Toxic Exposures

The delicate balance of neurotransmitter signaling may be disrupted by exposure to neurotoxic elements or chemicals. Life in modern society ensures daily exposure to a variety of neuroactive and neurotoxic substances. Exposure to toxicants may:

- induce epigenetic changes

- alter enzyme functions

- exhaust anti-oxidant reserves

- overwhelm detoxification pathways

Behavior changes in humans may occur for a variety of reasons, and toxicant exposures are known to induce behavior changes in humans (behavioral toxicity). Observing behavior changes in animals is a routine part of the assessment of potentially toxic substances. The neurotoxicity of many substances such as methyl mercury, lead and manganese were originally identified not because of their observed effects on laboratory animals, but because their adverse effects on human brain function have been well-documented in historical accounts.

Urinary neurotransmitters are being used to evaluate workers exposed to toxic chemicals and elements. A 2006 study of welders exposed to manganese demonstrated cognitive and behavioral changes along with decreased levels of urinary serotonin metabolites

A 2012 study demonstrated that workers exposed to the combustion product benzo[a]pyrene, when compared to unexposedworkers, had altered levels of urinary norepinephrine, dopamine, serotonin, and serotonin metabolites in addition to changes in learning and memory functions. A 2015 study of workers exposed to PCBs demonstrated alterations in neurotransmitter metabolites and cognitive functions when compared to unexposed workers.

The response to a toxic environmental exposure depends on an individual's:

- enzyme function
- detoxification capacity
- nutritional status
- cumulative toxic exposure load
- inheritance
- epigenetic influences (changes in DNA expression induced by the environment)

A variety of toxic environmental exposures may occur throughout life. Examples of more common potential toxic exposures are reviewed; symptoms and toxic effects often depend upon an individual's inheritance, nutritional status, detoxification capacity and cumulative toxic exposure history.

- Elements: Nutrients and Toxicants
  - **Nutrient elements,** such as copper and manganese are essential nutrients. They are cofactors for enzymes; deficiencies in nutrient elements may impair enzyme function. Deficiencies of nutrient elements may inhibit normal enzyme functions and physiology. However, in excess, nutrient elements may have toxic effects.

- **Copper** is essential for neurotransmitter synthesis, and plays a role in nervous system development. Excess copper may cause oxidative stress in the brain and body. Elevated copper levels have been associated with depression, irritability, learning disabilities and behavior disorders. Dysregulation of copper metabolism may contribute to the development of neurodegenerative diseases such as Alzheimer's disease, amyotrophic lateral sclerosis, Huntington disease, Menke's disease and Parkinson's disease.
- **Iodine** deficiency may result in neurological symptoms of depression.
- **Iron** deficiency may result in neurological symptoms of fatigue, irritability, and restless leg syndrome.
- **Lithium** may be neuroprotective. In excess, has been associated with neurological symptoms of confusion, tremor and slurred speech.
- **Magnesium** deficiency may result in neurological symptoms of muscular tremor or twitching, depression (possibly with psychosis), and if the deficiency is severe, convulsions.
- **Manganese**, chronic, subacute manganese exposure may result in late stage symptoms including speech disorders, abnormal gait, balance problems, and slow, clumsy movements. Final stage symptoms include gait

changes, tremor and chorea. Elevated levels of manganese may contribute to Parkinson's disease-like symptoms. Even low-level overexposure may alter motor functions, memory and mood, and may increase aggressive tendencies.

– **Phosphorus** deficiency may result in neurological symptoms of fatigue, paresthesias (tingling or burning skin sensations) and confusion.

– **Potassium** deficiency may result in neurological symptoms of fatigue and muscle weakness. Elevated potassium levels may contribute to symptoms of confusion, weakness, peripheral neuropathy and paresthesias.

– **Selenium** deficiency may exacerbate the effects of cadmium, mercury or arsenic exposure and bioaccumulation. Elevated levels of selenium may contribute to neurological symptoms of weakness and headache.

– **Vanadium** excess may contribute to neurological symptoms such as fatigue, vertigo, tremor, poor cognition and depression.

– **Zinc** deficiency may result in neurological symptoms such as apathy, fatigue, dysgeusia (altered taste perception) and loss of smell. Zinc deficiency may contribute to the progression of neurodegenerative diseases such as Parkinson's and Alzheimer's disease. Excess zinc may contribute to neurological symptoms such as fatigue, lethargy, dizziness and loss of fine motor skills such as difficulty writing.

Nutrient elements may be assessed by laboratory testing. More information about these tests is available at *www. doctorsdata.com.*

Red Blood Cell (RBC) Elements

Whole Blood Chromium & Vanadium

Urine Iodine

■ **Toxic Elements**, such as aluminum, arsenic, cadmium, lead and mercury, are so common in modern society that "acceptable" background levels of exposure have been established for many. Lead, in particular, is associated with developmental disorders, cognitive deficits and behavior problems. Toxic elements may competitively exclude nutrient elements from enzyme interactions. Many enzymes depend on mineral co-factors for proper function, and the replacement of a nutrient mineral element with a toxic element may inhibit enzyme function. A complete overview of symptoms related to toxic element exposures may be found at the Agency for Toxic Substances and Disease Registry (ATSDR) at *http://www.atsdr.cdc. gov/.* The symptoms reviewed here relate more to chronic background exposure and bioaccumulation than symptoms of acute poisoning. Many toxic elements may have cumulative and synergistic effects at low levels of exposure.

- **Aluminum** has neurotoxic effects as high levels of exposure and bioaccumulation. Early neurological symptoms may include fatigue, anxiety, irritability, numbness, weakness and headache. Neurons are susceptible to long-term accumulation. Bioaccumulation of aluminum may be associated with pre-senile dementia and Alzheimer's disease.
- **Antimony** exposure may induce neurologic symptoms of fatigue and headache.
- **Arsenic** exposures may result in a variety of neurologic symptoms, including fatigue and peripheral neuropathy from chronic, subacute exposures (bioaccumulation).
- **Barium** exposure at chronic high levels (bioaccumulation) may contribute to sensory neuropathy and loss of tendon reflexes.
- **Bromide** exposure and bioaccumulation may result in neurological symptoms. At high levels, symptoms of headache, fatigue, ataxia, and memory loss have been reported.
- **Cadmium** bioaccumulation may contribute to peripheral neuropathy.
- **Cesium** in cerebrospinal fluid has been associated with brain tumors, and neurodegenerative diseases such as Amyotrophic lateral sclerosis (ALS) and motor neuron disease. Cesium may block glycine receptors in the nervous system. Peripheral neuropathy may occur if high levels of exposure occur; seizures have been reported.
- **Chromium** elevations have been reported in patients with cerebral hemorrhage and stroke. Unsupervised supplementation has resulted in insomnia and unpleasant dream activity in some individuals.
- **Fluoride** is neurotoxic at high levels; exposure may affect children's developing brains. Recent studies indicate that fluoride exposure may impair cognitive functions and learning.
- **Germanium** is reported to be neurotoxic.
- **Lead** has been associated with developmental and behavior disorders in children at relatively low levels of exposure; there may be no safe level of lead exposure. Other neurological symptoms, of low IQ, hearing loss and poor coordination, have also been reported. Higher levels of lead exposure have been associated with other neurological symptoms, including decreased nerve action potential, tremors, neuropathies, encephalopathy (global brain dysfunction) and neurotoxicity.
- **Mercury** exposure symptoms may vary based on the chemical form of the mercury and exposure history to other toxic elements or chemicals. Neurological symptoms of mercury exposure include headaches, decreased sensory perception, fatigue, peripheral neuropathy, neuromuscular

disorders, memory and cognitive deficits.
- **Tellurium** exposure at high levels resulted in neurologic symptoms of impaired learning and spatial memory (animal studies).
- **Thallium** bioaccumulation may result in neurological symptoms including mental confusion, fatigue, paresthesias, myalgias, tremor and ataxia (motor incoordination). High levels of exposure may result in additional symptoms of optic neuritis, sleep disturbance, and possibly psychosis.
- **Tin** exposure and bioaccumulation may contribute to neurological symptoms including loss of smell, headaches, fatigue, ataxia and vertigo.
- **Uranium exposure** of 1mg/kg in animals resulted in neurological symptoms of decreased activity, decreased forelimb grip and impaired working memory. Levels of the neurotransmitter dopamine were decreased by 30% during uranium exposure.

Toxic elements may be assessed by laboratory testing. More information about these tests is available at *www.doctorsdata.com*.

Toxic and Essential Elements Testing

Red Blood Cell (RBC) Elements

Urine Halides

- Toxic chemicals
  Renewed interest in neurotoxicity was initiated in the 1970s when Danish, Finnish, and Swedish investigators reported an increased frequency of neuropsychiatric symptoms and signs of impaired performance during neurobehavioural tests. The evaluations were given to painters, laquerers, printers, jet fuel exposure and other chemically exposed industrial workers. The workers experienced reduced vigilance, decreased response time memory and cognition changes Other organic chemicals, such as styrene, have also been associated with behavior changes in exposed workers. Toxic chemicals may be inhaled, ingested or absorbed across the skin. Pesticides solvents, and polycyclic aromatic hydrocarbons (PAHs) are some of the main chemical groups that are recognized for health problem caused by dermal absorption Background chemical exposure of the general population occurs daily due to chemicals ingested in food or water, or inhaled as volatile organic compounds (VOCs) Chemical exposures may be greater for those living in industrial areas, near waste disposal facilities or hazardous waste sites.

Chemicals are classified by their structure and properties chemicals in the same class tend to have similar effects. Individual responses to any toxic exposure will depend on a variety of factors including age, route of exposure nutritional status, inheritance, detoxification capacity and history of other toxic exposures. Animal studies indicate that some chemical exposure effects may be transient, and resolve after exposure as the chemical is metabolized

The effects of chemical exposures may be additive and synergistic, and chemical effects may be additive and synergistic with the effects of toxic elements.

There is very little information on the human bioaccumulation of many toxic chemicals. However, persistent organic pollutants (POPs), can remain in the environment for years, even decades, without degrading. In general, fat soluble chemical compounds more easily cross the blood brain barrier (BBB) and may be stored in body fat. The ability to detoxify and metabolize chemicals may be compromised by age, nutritional status, disease or inheritance.

For additional information about any chemical class or for further information about specific chemicals, the following resources are available:

– Agency for Toxic Substances and Disease Registry (ATSDR) at *http://www. atsdr.cdc.gov/substances/ ToxChemicalClasses.asp*
– National Institute of Health ToxNet *http://toxnet.nlm.nih. gov/*
– National Report on Human Exposure to Environmental Chemicals from the Centers for Disease Control and Prevention (CDC) *http:// www.cdc.gov/exposurereport/*
– Information about contaminants found at hazardous waste sites *http:// www.atsdr.cdc.gov/toxprofiles/ index.asp*
– Information about indoor environmental air quality

from the CDC *http://www. cdc.gov/niosh/topics/indoorenv/ ChemicalsOdors.html*

In addition to toxic metals and manufactured chemicals, a variety of other exposures may affect neurotransmitters and neurological function:

• Chronic **alcohol** consumption has been associated with an increased incidence of a variety of diseases, including central nervous system (CNS) degeneration. Neurological symptoms of heavy alcohol use may include dementia, impaired cognition and impaired motor functions. Alcohol consumption may increase acetalaldehyde levels and oxidative stress in the brain. Adolescents engaged in binge drinking behaviors show poorer cognitive performance and altered patterns of gray and white brain matter.

• **Nicotine**, found in tobacco products, is a neuro-active substance that activates acetylcholine nicotinic receptors. A recent study has documented that smoking may contribute to the thinning of the brain's cortex. Cortical thinning has been associated with aging, cognitive decline and dementia.

• **Naturally occurring toxins** may be found in plants, algae and fungi. The toxins may bioaccumulate in the animals that ingest the plants or fungi.
  ▪ **Alkaloids** are a class of organic compounds that may have obvious physiological effects. Alkaloid compounds may be active ingredients in pharmaceuticals, such as morphine and quinine. Alkaloids may be found in over 4,000

plant species, and in some fungi, such as the ergot fungus *Claviceps*. A class of alkaloids, beta-carboline alkaloids, have been associated with increased incidence of essential tremor and neurodegenerative disorders. Harmane, one of the best-studied beta-carbolines, is found in meats, fish, coffee and cigarettes. There is evidence that harmane may be absorbed directly into the bloodstream, bypassing the liver. Harmane is soluble in fats, which allows it to cross the blood brain barrier. Elevated levels in the central nervous system have been associated with essential tremor and neurodegenerative diseases.

■ Harmful Algae Blooms (HABs) may contaminate fish with neurotoxins. Symptoms usually disappear in a few days or weeks, but in some people the neurotoxin is not metabolized and neurologic symptoms may last for years. Algal neurotoxins may be difficult to identify.

– The most common type of algal neurotoxin, ciguatera, may be found in barracuda, black grouper, blackfin snapper, cubera snapper, dog snapper, greater amberjack, hogfish, horse-eye jack, king mackerel, and yellowfin grouper. Neurological symptoms of ciguatera include weakness; headache; numbness, tingling, burning sensations around the mouth, hands, or feet; reversal of temperature sensation in the mouth (cold things feel hot and hot things feel cold); unusual taste sensations; nightmares; or hallucinations.

Ciguatera is detoxified by cytochrome P450 enzymes.

– Domoic acid is a neurotoxin produced by a diatom. Domoic acid bioaccumulates in the fish and shellfish that eat the diatoms. The neurotoxin causes kidney damage, and domoic acid poisoning is known to have lethal effects on marine mammals. In humans the toxin causes amnesiac shellfish poisoning (ASP) and neurological symptoms include headaches, vertigo, confusion, disorientation, short-term memory loss, motor weakness, seizures and coma. Symptoms usually begin within 48 hours of seafood consumption.

• **Lipopolysaccharides** and peptidoglycans from gastrointestinal bacteria, if released into the circulation, may contribute to neural inflammation in the central nervous system and may downregulate liver phase I detoxification. (See **Digestion and Absorption** section.)

• **Allergy** sensitization may contribute to neurological symptoms. Food allergy has been associated with anxiety and depression symptoms in patients. In animal models sensitized mice were orally challenged with allergen and demonstrated increased levels of anxiety. Human studies demonstrate that plasma levels of serotonin may be elevated in symptomatic asthmatic patients.

Detoxification

One of the liver's primary functions is the detoxification of xenobiotics (foreign compounds) so they may be excreted in urine or bile. Three phases of detoxification occur:

- Phase I detoxification occurs as cytochrome P450, oxidase, reductase and dehydrogenase enzymes add a hydroxyl group (-OH) onto organic compounds. This step converts fat-soluble compounds into water-soluble compounds.

  - Toxic metals such as arsenic, cadmium, mercury and lead may inhibit cytochrome P450 enzymes. More information about these tests is available at *www.doctorsdata.com.*

    #### Urine Toxic Metals

    #### Whole Blood Elements

    - Heme is incorporated into all cytochrome P450 enzymes
    - Heme is synthesized by the porphyrin pathway. The porphyrin pathway may be evaluated in the laboratory. More information about this test is available at *www.doctorsdata.com.*

      #### Urine Porphyrins

  - Xenobiotics activated by phase I may generate reactive oxygen species and increase oxidative stress
  - Lipopolysaccharides and peptidoglycans from gastrointestinal bacteria, if released into the circulation may contribute to neural inflammation in the central nervous system and may downregulate liver phase I detoxification. (See **Digestion and Absorption** section.) Digestion and absorption may be evaluated in the laboratory. More information about these tests is available at *www.doctorsdata.com.*

    #### Comprehensive Stool Analysis

    #### Intestinal Permeability

    - Nutrients that may support phase I include selenium, zinc and vitamins A, D, E, K, and C. Plant compounds, such as sulforaphanes found in broccoli and other Brassica family vegetables also support detoxification. More information about this test is available at *www.doctorsdata.com.*

      #### Red Blood Cell (RBC) Elements

- Phase II detoxification occurs through a variety of different reactions including glucuronidation, sulfation, methylation, N-acetylation, and conjugation with amino acids or the attachment of glutathione.

  - Phase II conjugation may be inhibited by arsenic, cadmium, lead, mercury and hexavalant chromium which inhibit the enzyme glutathione S-transferase (GST).

    - An isoform of GST found in neurons prevents neurodegeneration.

  - Glutathione (GSH) needs to be available for the GST enzyme to function; low levels of GSH may occur if synthesis is compromised by enzyme defects or if there are enzyme defects in

the methylation pathway. (See **Methylation** section.)
  - GSH is the primary antioxidant in the body. Low levels predispose cells towards oxidative stress. Oxidative stress is a contributing factor to neurodegeneration.
- Nutrients that may support phase II include reduced glutathione, N-acetyl cysteine (glutathione precursor), B vitamins and calcium-D-glucarate
  - The amino acids glutamine, glycine, and taurine are used in Phase II conjugation

• Phase III detoxification occurs when the metabolized xenobiotic is transported out of the cell for excretion in urine or bile. Phase III efflux pumps require ATP. Nutrients that may support phase III include B vitamins, magnesium, manganese, iron, and CoQ10. More information about this test is available at *www. doctorsdata.com.*

Red Blood Cell (RBC) Elements

A diet rich in fruits, vegetables and healthy (omega-3) fats will also support liver functions. Liver phase I and II functions, oxidative stress, methylation pathway capability and glutathione levels may all be evaluated in the laboratory. More information about these tests is available at *www.doctorsdata.com.*

Hepatic Detox Profile

DNA Oxidative Damage Assay

Methylation Profile; plasma

Glutathione; erythrocytes

A Functional Approach to Neurotransmission

While not every neurological dysfunction may be completely reversed by dietary changes, detoxification and the nutritional support of biochemical enzyme pathways, a great many obstacles to optimum function may be removed by these therapies. Bredesen (2014) in a pilot study with ten patients suffering from Alzheimer's and other types of dementia, memory and cognitive dysfunctions, has outlined a functional approach that may slow neurodegeneration and minimize oxidative stress in the brain. Eight of the ten subjects improved sufficiently to return to work or kept working with improved performance. The results are suggestive that the early stages of cognitive decline may be exacerbated by metabolic dysregulation. Bredesen suggests that the basic tenets of the individualized programs may be used to minimize metabolic dysregulation, inflammation and oxidative stress that may contribute to neurodegeneration and neurological symptoms; the need for many of the suggested interventions may be evaluated in the laboratory:

• Elimination of simple carbohydrates to minimize inflammation and insulin resistance
  - **Metabolomic Profile**

• Fast 12 hours each night, including 3 hours prior to bedtime to reduce insulin levels and decrease amyloid-formation

• Exercise 30-60 minutes 4-6 days weekly

• Normalize homocysteine levels
  - **Plasma Methylation Profile**
  - **DNA Methylation Pathway**

- Maintain serum B12 > 500
- Normalize inflammatory biomarkers with anti-inflammatory diet, curcumin, omega-3 fatty acids
  - Fatty Acids; Erythrocytes
- Normalize and optimize thyroid and other hormone levels
  - Thyroid Profile
- Promote gastrointestinal health; optimize digestion and absorption; eliminate inflammation and minimize autoimmunity; promote health of gastrointestinal microbiome
  - Comprehensive Stool Analysis
  - Intestinal Permeability
- Normalize vitamin D levels
  - Vitamin D Serum or Bloodspot
- Optimize antioxidant status with nutrients such as mixed tocopherols and tocotrienols (Vitamin E), selenium, α-lipoic acid, vitamin C, antioxidant foods such as blueberries
  - Red Blood Cell (RBC) Elements
- Optimize mitochondrial function with nutrients such as CoQ10, α-lipoic acid, acetyl-L-carnitine, selenium, zinc, resveratrol, vitamin C, thiamine (B1)

  - Red Blood Cell (RBC) Elements
- Increase focus with pantothenic acid (B5) required for acetylcholine synthesis
- Enhance NAD-dependent protein deacetylase sirtuin-1 (SirT1) function with resveratrol and zinc
  - Red Blood Cell (RBC) Elements
- Assess toxic element exposure and detoxify
  - Hair Elements
  - Urine Toxic Metals
  - Whole Blood Elements
- Optimize sleep and rule out sleep apnea to reduce cortisol releasing factor and cortisol

  - A recent animal study has revealed a dopamine-regulated "ultradian" biorhythm of approximately four hours, that, when disregulated, may contribute to perturbed sleep-wake cycles commonly seen in neuropsychiatric disorders. Early evidence indicates that structured mealtimes and bedtimes may provide additional, alternate biorhythm cues to help maintain ultradian and circadian rhythms.

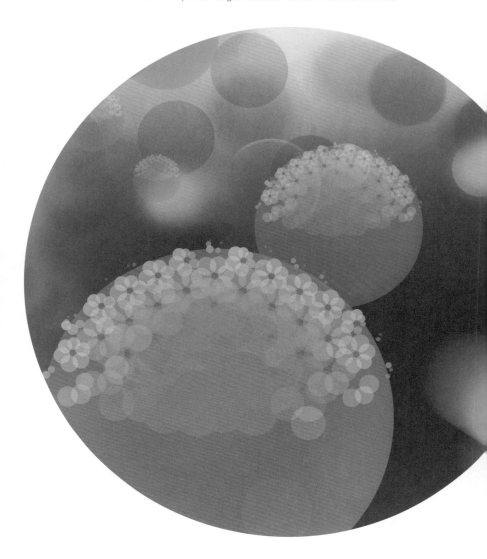

Neurotransmitter Analytes:

Dopamine

The catecholamine, dopamine (DA), plays a primary role in the control of motor, cognitive, behavioral (emotional) and endocrine functions in the central nervous system (CNS). Dopamine nerve pathways in the brain affect voluntary movements, feeding, behavioral affect, emotion, reward signaling, attention, speech, memory, learning and sleep. Too much or too little dopamine may affect memory and cognition. Dopamine signaling controls hormone release from the anterior pituitary gland. Dopamine serves as a neurotransmitter in the CNS, in the adrenal glands, and in autocrine/paracrine signalling throughout the body. Dopamine is an important regulator of systemic blood pressure and gastrointestinal functions. Impairment in the central dopamine pathways and metabolism has been suggested as a factor in the pathogenesis of restless leg syndrome (RLS). Animal studies indicate that dopamine release in the brain correlates to the calorie load of food ingested or infused into the gastrointestinal tract. Dopamine signaling also affects the retina, sense of smell and hormone status.

Dopamine may also function as a neuromodulator, as dopamine modulates calcium signaling. The flow of calcium and other ions into and out of neurons changes the action potential within the nerve. Dopamine is an inhibitory neurotransmitter and dopamine calcium signaling may be the mechanism that counteracts the damaging effects of excess glutamate (excitotoxicity) in the brain.

Dopamine signaling contributes to motivated behavior. Animal studies indicate that different areas of the brain are involved in different aspects of motivational activity (such as feeding) and reward behavior. Dopamine signaling may play a role in addictive behaviors; drugs such as cocaine and amphetamine have been shown to increase dopamine concentrations in nerve synapses. Disregulation of dopamine signaling has been associated schizophrenia, attention deficit, and neurodegenerative diseases such as Parkinson's.

Effects:

Decreased dopamine release in the motor pathway, or a dysfunction of dopamine receptors, leads to movement disorders. The loss of dopamine neurons is associated with neurodegenerative disorders such as Parkinson's disease, and results in motor symptoms such as rigidity, tremor or bradykinesia (slow movement). Oxidative stress and mitochondrial dysfunction are common causes of neurodegeneration. Low dopamine levels have been associated with depression, apathy, fatigue, low pain tolerance and decreased sense of pleasure (hypohedonia). Difficulty concentrating, loss of libido, obesity, cold extremities, muscle weakness and lowered body temperature may occur. Decreased Dopamine production or signaling has been associated with attention deficit hyperactivity disorder (ADHD), social anxiety and GTP cyclohydrolase 1 deficiency (Segawa Disease). Experiments have shown that various patterns of dopamine/receptor bindings alter T-cell differentiation and behavior, and may contribute to autoimmune and inflammatory reactions in the body and the CNS. Adult phenlyketonuria patients with low dopamine levels report symtoms of drastic mood swings, difficulty paying attention, and sleep disturbances.

Copper is associated, directly or indirectly with several neurological diseases, including Parkinson's and Alzheimer disease. Enzymes in the CNS rely on copper cofactors, including dopamine-β-hydoxylase (DβH) and tyrosinase (melanocytes). Manganese excess is associated with Parkinson's-like symptoms. Tyrosine hydrolase function may be affected by oxidative stress, nitrosative stress and thiolation. Metyrosine therapy which decreases the activity of tyrosine hydroxylase will decrease dopamine levels. Tyrosine supplements may decrease urinary excretion of dopamine.

Excess dopamine activity in the brain leads to stereotyped behaviors in experimental animals and may account for some of the symptoms of schizophrenia. (Current research indicates that excess neurotransmitter or receptor function in both dopamine and serotonin pathways may contribute to schizophrenia.) Elevated dopamine levels may affect behavior and have been associated with obsessive-compulsive disorder (OCD), Attention Deficit Disorders (ADD), impulsivity, addictive behavior, schizophrenia and other psychiatric disorders. Research continues to determine if elevated dopamine or impaired dopamine receptors are the causative agents. Stressful stimuli have been shown to increase dopamine release.

Dopamine's action on the pituitary gland leads to reduced prolactin and increased growth hormone release. Dopamine signals vasodilatation of blood vessels in the kidney and mesentery artery through interaction with dopamine receptors; but signals vasoconstriction elsewhere via β1-adrenoceptors. It stimulates the heart via β1-adrenoceptors. Elevated urinary dopamine in adults has been associated with drug effects and physiologic conditions including pheochromocytoma, carcinoid tumor and pregnancy. Elevations in children have been associated with physiologic conditions such as neuroblastoma, Costello syndrome, leukemia, pheochromocytoma, Menke's disease and rhabdomyosarcoma of the bladder. Dopamine, and drugs that mimic it, may cause nausea and vomiting through an action on a trigger zone in the brain stem. Administration of L-DOPA medications will elevate urinary dopamine levels.

Decreased function or blockage of N-methyl-D-aspartate (NMDA) glutamate receptors may contribute to psychotic symptoms. Reduced glutamate signaling has been associated with elevations in dopamine and may contribute to symptoms of schizophrenia.

Synthesis and Metabolism:

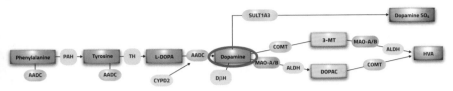

Dopamine is synthesized in the CNS, in the adrenal glands, and in various peripheral organs. The biosynthesis of dopamine begins with the hydroxylation of tyrosine by tyrosine hydroxylase (TH) to form the precursor 3,4-dihydroxyphenylalanine (L-DOPA). Tyrosine hydroxylation is normally tightly regulated, and requires tetrahydrobiopterin and iron co-factors. Tyrosine hydroxylase is located in dopamine and norepinephrine neurons in various brain areas. In the periphery, TH is found in the adrenal medulla and in sympathetic ganglia (nerve clusters). Animal studies indicate that selenium-deficient diets increase the activity of tyrosine hydroxylase twofold. Selenium deficiency also decreased the expression of glutathione peroxidase and glutathione reductase; decreased expression of these enzymes may increase intracellular oxidative stress. TH enzyme function may be downregulated by oxidative stress, nitrosative stress and thiolation (reactions with sulfur amino acids). Single nucleotide polymorphisms (SNPs) in the genes coding for tyrosine hydroxylase have been associated with altered stress responses, blood pressure, heart rate and norepinephrine secretion.

Dopamine, norepinephrine, and epinephrine are all feedback inhibitors of tyrosine hydroxylase (TH), which synthesizes 3,4-dihydroxyphenylalanine (L-DOPA). L-DOPA is then de-carboxyated by aromatic amino acid decarboxylase (AADC). Excess manganese may interfere with catecholamine metabolism in the adrenal glands; it also decreases tetrahydrobiopterin levels. In vitro studies indicate that exposure to high levels of manganese decreases dopamine metabolite levels.

Aromatic amino acid decarboxylase (AADC) activity is dependent on dopamine levels, but not specific to dopamine. AADC requires pyridoxal phosphate (vitamin B6) as a cofactor. The enzyme also metabolizes tyrosine, tryptophan and histidine as well. Increased dopamine levels increase AADC activity, which may then affect other neurotransmitter levels. Once synthesized, dopamine is sequestered into synaptic vesicles by the vesicular monoamine transporter (VMAT2). Storing dopamine inside vesicles prevents oxidative stress to the cytosol of neurons. Vesicle storage may be disrupted by reserpine, amphetamines, or similar compounds. Mutations or SNPs in VMAT2 may also affect the ability of cell to sequester neurotransmitters. Animal and in vitro studies have also demonstrated dopamine synthesis from cytochrome P450 enzymes (CYP450). In this pathway, tyrosine is first converted to tyramine, which is then hydroxylated by CYPD2 enzymes. This pathway may be used in the CNS and the peripheral nervous system to synthesize dopamine, research continues in this area.

Almost half the dopamine synthesized in the body is found in the gastrointestinal tract (GIT). GIT mucosal cells produce either dopamine or its receptors. Evidence indicates that conversion of circulating L-DOPA to dopamine in the kidney may accounts for the majority of the free dopamine in urine. DDI measures the free fraction of urinary neurotransmitters; approximately 20% of urinary dopamine is free (unconjugated). Dopamine synthesized in the kidney is necessary for the maintenance of normal blood pressure and renal function. Renal excretion of dopamine may decrease in cases of heart failure. Studies in hypertensive patients indicate that sodium excretion correlates with urinary free dopamine excretion. Animal studies indicate that intra-renal dopamine deficiency may contribute to hypertension and decreased longevity.

Extracellular dopamine has to be removed from the synaptic cleft to stop neuron activation. It can either be recycled after reuptake by the dopamine transporter (DAT). Defects in DAT function may arise from mutations or single nucleotide polymorphisms (SNPs) in the DNA that codes for the DAT enzyme. Alterations in DAT function may contribute to Alzheimer's disease (with parkinsonism), schizophrenia, and Tourette's syndrome, Wilson's disease and Lesch-Nyhan disease. DAT function may also decrease with age.

Dopamine is converted into norepinephrine by dopamine β-hydroxylase (DβH). DβH requires copper and vitamin C as cofactors. Dopamine may also be degraded by intraneuronal monoamine oxidase (MAO) and extraneuronal catechol-O methyl transferase (COMT). MAO has two different isoforms, encoded on two different genes, MAO-A and MAO-B. Both enzyme

forms oxidize dopamine; the MAO isoforms vary by brain region. MAO-B is the predominant isoform in the glial cells. MAO converts dopamine to DOPAC. MAO-B may be inhibited by cigarette smoke. Excess phenylethylamine (PEA) may be the only clue to monoamine oxidase B (MAO-B) deficiency. Animal studies indicate that the addition of selenium and tocopherols to the diet may increase antioxidant capacity and decrease MAO-B activity. Forskolin increases plasma DOPAC levels in animals. COMT uses S-adenosyl-methionine (SAM) and a magnesium cofactor to degrade dopamine into 3-methoxytyramine (3-MT). MAOA and COMT further convert the intermediary metabolites to homovanilic acid (HVA), the final metabolite. Dopamine and its metabolites may be further conjugated by liver phase II reactions prior to excretion. Pre-synaptic uptake and metabolism of dopamine give rise to 3,4-dihydroxyphenylacetic acid (DOPAC), a different metabolite. Post-synaptic uptake and metabolism produced both DOPAC and 3-MT.

Oxidative deamination by MAO produces hydrogen peroxide and a reactive aldehyde, which may increase oxidative stress and use up the cell's glutathione pool. Aldehyde dehydrogenase (ALDH) converts aldehydes to fatty acids. Two dopamine intermediaries may elevate and have neurotoxic effects (increased oxidative stress) if ALDH function is compromised. AADC activity is dependent on dopamine levels; poor MAO function may inhibit AADC activity, which may further increase dopamine levels. The COMT reaction depends on the availability of S-adenosyl-methionine (SAM), which regenerates from homocysteine by cobalamin-dependent methylation from 5-methyltetrahydrofolate.

COMT methylation of catecholamines may exhaust a cell's methylation capacity. Excess DOPA from medications may increase oxidative stress from MAO and COMT catabolism and contribute to increased homocysteine levels and peripheral neuropathies. High levels of iron may further increase oxidative stress in the CNS.

Sulfotransferase (SULT)1A3 catalyzes the sulfate conjugation of dopamine. There are two SULT1A3 genes which may be expressed and active; this will affect individual variations in enzyme activity. SULT1A3 converts dopamine to dopamine sulfate, which is excreted in the urine. Sulfotransferase (SULT) enzymes are not found in neurons. SULT activity has been down-regulated in vitro by coffee compounds, green tea polyphenols, quercitin and resveratrol. SULT enzymes also conjugate a variety of xenobiotic chemicals that may be inhaled or ingested during environmental exposures. Elevated levels of metanephrine and normetanephrine may indicate SULT deficiency.

Inheritance may affect dopamine synthesis and metabolism, dopamine receptor function, stress-induced dopamine release. Single nucleotide polymorphisms (SNPs) in dopamine- and oxytocin-related genes have been shown to alter stress-induced dopamine release. Enzyme deficiencies may be inherited or acquired from nutritional deficiency or toxicant exposure.

Receptors

Dopamine activates dopamine receptors D_1-D_5. Dopamine receptors are expressed at different densities in the CNS. The neurotransmitter, bound to its receptor, is the active, functional unit. There are many dopamine re-

ceptor subtypes in the brain that affect behavior, attention, impulse control, decisions, sleep, and reproductive behaviors. Most neurons and peripheral cells possess receptors for multiple types of neurotransmitters, and the final cellular response may be the result of multiple simultaneous signals. Neurotransmitter receptors are often the targets of pharmaceuticals designed to stimulate or inhibit dopamine signaling. Dopamine receptor signaling may affect the behavior of N-type calcium channels (and other ionotropic receptors), NMDA receptors, and GABA-A receptors. Intracellular signaling pathways affected by dopamine receptors are important in regulating cell cycles, cell proliferation and homeostasis.

Genetic mutations or SNPs in the DNA coding for receptor structure may affect dopamine receptor functions. In the CNS, alterations in D_2 receptor expression and CNS density have been associated with Parkinson's disease; altered D_1 density has been reported as systems atrophy progresses. Altered D_1 and D_2 expression has been associated with Huntington's disease. SNPs in D_2, D_3, and D_4 receptors have been associated with schizophrenia and treatment responses. No changes in dopamine receptor expression or CNS density have currently been associated with Alzheimer's dementia.

D_1 receptors

- Motor activity, reward, learning, memory (working memory), renin secretion, renal function, blood pressure, vasodilation, gastrointestinal motility

- Stimulates adenylate cyclase

- Modulates NMDA receptor functions

- Chronic blockade of D_2 receptors may downregulate D_1 receptor expression and affect working memory
- Animal studies associate D_1 receptor functions with fear responses, aversion behaviors, grooming, maternal, mating and memory
- Animal studies indicate that overstimulation of D_1 receptors may predispose neurons to epigenetic insults

D_2 receptors

- Motor activity, reward, learning, memory, sympathetic tone, prolactin secretion, aldosterone secretion, renal function, blood pressure, vasodilation, gastrointestinal motility
- May have autoreceptor functions
- Inhibits adenylate cyclase
- Chronic blockade of D_2 receptors may downregulate D_1 receptor expression and affect working memory
- Mutations in the DRD_2 gene have been associated with myoclonic dystonia
- Genetic variations in DRD_2 (paternal and grandpaternal transmission) may influence susceptibility to alcoholism
- D_2 antagonist medications have anti-psychotic effects.

D_3 receptors

- Motor activity, reward, cognitive, modulate D_2
- Genetic variations in DRD_3 may be associated with hereditary essential tremor disorder

D_4 receptors

- Cognitive, renal function, blood pressure, vasodilation, gastrointestinal motility
- Found in mesolimbic system of brain that regulates emotion and complex behavior
- Contributes to regulation of circadian rhythms

D_5 (1B) receptors

- Cognitive
- Genetic variations may be associated with autosomal dominant cervical (neck) dystonia and benign essential blepharospasm

Consider:

Tyrosine on an empty stomach may improve transport across BBB; may be contraindicated in hypertension; may induce anxiety in some patients.

Further evaluations:

- Essential precursor Amino Acid status (**Plasma** or **Urine Amino Acids**)
- Magnesium status (**RBC Elements**)
- Iron status (**RBC Elements**)
- Copper status (**RBC Elements**)
- Manganese status (**RBC Elements**)
- Selenium status (**RBC Elements**)
- Glutathione status (**Glutathione; erythrocytes**)
- Oxidative stress (**DNA Oxidative Damage Assay/8-OHdG**)
- Methylation pathway activity (**Plasma Methylation Profile, DNA Methylation Pathway**)
- Toxicant exposures (**Urine Toxic Elements**)

References:

Bannon, Michael J., Sacchetti, Paola, and Granneman, James G.
The Dopamine Transporter: Potential Involvement in Neuropsychiatric Disorders
Neuropsychopharmacology: The Fifth Generation of Progress
Lippincott, Williams, & Wilkins, Philadelphia, Pennsylvania, 2002

Beaulieu, Jean-Martin; Gainetdinov, Raul R. (2011)
The Physiology, Signaling, and Pharmacology of Dopamine Receptors
Pharmacol. Rev. vol. 63 (1) p. 182-217

Bromek, Ewa; Haduch, Anna; Gołembiowska, Krystyna; Daniel, Władysława A (2011)
Cytochrome P450 mediates dopamine formation in the brain in vivo.
Journal of neurochemistry vol. 118 (5) p. 806-15

Buttarelli, Francesca R; Fanciulli, Alessandra; Pellicano, Clelia; Pontieri, Francesco E (2011)
The dopaminergic system in peripheral blood lymphocytes: from physiology to pharmacology and potential applications to neuropsychiatric disorders.
Current neuropharmacology vol. 9 (2) p. 278-88

Castaño, A; Ayala, A; Rodriguez-Gomez, J A; de la Cruz, C P; Revilla, E et al. (1995)
Increase in dopamine turnover and tyrosine hydroxylase enzyme in hippocampus of rats fed on low selenium diet.
Journal of neuroscience research vol. 42 (5) p. 684-91

Coughtrie, Michael W. H.; Johnston, Laura E. (2001)
Interactions between Dietary Chemicals and Human Sulfotransferases{---}Molecular Mechanisms and Clinical Significance
Drug Metab. Dispos. vol. 29 (4) p. 522-528

de Araujo, Ivan E; Ferreira, Jozélia G; Tellez, Luis A; Ren, Xueying; Yeckel, Catherine W (2012)
The gut-brain dopamine axis: a regulatory system for caloric intake.
Physiology & behavior vol. 106 (3) p. 394-9

Eisenhofer, Graeme; Kopin, Irwin J.; Goldstein, David S. (2004)
Catecholamine Metabolism: A Contemporary View with Implications for Physiology and Medicine
Pharmacol. Rev. vol. 56 (3) p. 331-349

Ferreira, António; Bettencourt, Paulo; Pestana, Manuel; Correia, Flora; Serrão, Paula et al. (2001)
Heart failure, aging, and renal synthesis of dopamine
American Journal of Kidney Diseases vol. 38 (3) p. 502-509

Glavin, Gary B.; Szabo, Sandor (1990)
Dopamine in gastrointestinal disease
Digestive Diseases and Sciences vol. 35 (9) p. 1153-1161

Love, Tiffany M; Enoch, Mary-Anne; Hodgkinson, Colin A; Peciña, Marta; Mickey, Brian et al. (2012)
Oxytocin gene polymorphisms influence human dopaminergic function in a sex-dependent manner.
Biological psychiatry vol. 72 (3) p. 198-206

Meiser, Johannes; Weindl, Daniel; Hiller, Karsten (2013)
Complexity of dopamine metabolism.
Cell communication and signaling : CCS vol. 11 (1) p. 34

National PKU Alliance
http://adultswithpku.org/Home.aspx
Accessed 23 January 2015

Nextprot Beta
DRD2>>D(2) dopamine receptor *http://www.nextprot.org/db/entry/NX_P14416/medical*
DRD3>>D(3) dopamine receptor *http://www.nextprot.org/db/entry/NX_P35462/medical*

DRD4>>D(4) dopamine receptor *http://www.nextprot.org/db/entry/NX_P21917*
DRD5>>D(1B) dopamine receptor *http://www.nextprot.org/db/entry/NX_P21918/medical*
Accessed 19 January 2015

Niwa, Toshiro; Hiroi, Toyoko; Tsuzuki, Daisuke; Yamamoto, Shigeo; Narimatsu, Shizuo et al. (2004)
Effect of genetic polymorphism on the metabolism of endogenous neuroactive substances, progesterone and p-tyramine, catalyzed by CYP2D6
Molecular Brain Research vol. 129 (1) p. 117-123

OMIM Online Mendelian Inheritance in Man
DOPAMINE RECEPTOR D1; DRD1 *http://omim.org/entry/126449 Accessed 19 January 2015*

Pehek, Elizabeth A; Nocjar, Christine; Roth, Bryan L; Byrd, Tara A; Mabrouk, Omar S (2005)
Evidence for the Preferential Involvement of 5-HT2A Serotonin Receptors in Stress- and Drug-Induced Dopamine Release in the Rat Medial Prefrontal Cortex
Neuropsychopharmacology (2006) 31, 265–277. doi:10.1038/sj.npp.1300819; published online 6 July 2005

Rasheed, Naila; Alghasham, Abdullah (2012)
Central dopaminergic system and its implications in stress-mediated neurological disorders and gastric ulcers: short review.
Advances in pharmacological sciences vol. 2012 p. 182671

Sistrunk, Shannon C; Ross, Matthew K; Filipov, Nikolay M (2007)
Direct effects of manganese compounds on dopamine and its metabolite Dopac: an in vitro study.
Environmental toxicology and pharmacology vol. 23 (3) p. 286-96

Trachte, George J; Uncini, Thomas; Hinz, Marty (2009)

Both stimulatory and inhibitory effects of dietary 5-hydroxytryptophan and tyrosine are found on urinary excretion of serotonin and dopamine in a large human population.
Neuropsychiatric disease and treatment vol. 5 p. 227-35

UniProt
P21728- DRD1_HUMAN
http://www.uniprot.org/uniprot/P21728
Accessed 19 January 2015

Vaarmann, A; Kovac, S; Holmström, K M; Gandhi, S; Abramov, A Y (2013)
Dopamine protects neurons against glutamate-induced excitotoxicity.
Cell death & disease vol. 4 p. e455

Zhang, Ming-Zhi; Yao, Bing; Wang, Suwan; Fan, Xiaofeng; Wu, Guanqing et al. (2011)
Intrarenal dopamine deficiency leads to hypertension and decreased longevity in mice.
The Journal of clinical investigation vol. 121 (7) p. 2845-54

Zhang, Yanrong; Cuevas, Santiago; Asico, Laureano D; Escano, Crisanto; Yang, Yu et al. (2012)
Deficient dopamine D2 receptor function causes renal inflammation independently of high blood pressure.
PloS one vol. 7 (6) p. e38745

3,4-Dihydroxyphenylacetic acid (DOPAC)

DOPAC, the major intermediate metabolite of dopamine, is found in neurons near the synaptic vesicles and in the extracellular space. Research indicates that approximately one-third of newly synthesized dopamine is immediately processed to DOPAC, which is then secreted into the extracellular spaces between neurons.

Effects:

Decreased levels of DOPAC have been associated with several conditions. Impairment in the central dopamine pathways and metabolism has been suggested as a factor in the pathogenesis of restless leg syndrome (RLS). DOPAC inhibits the fibrillation of a-synnuclein; the aggregation of alpha-synnuclein is associated with an increased risk of Parkinson's disease and other neurodegenerative disorders. The inhibition of a-synuclein induces oxidative stress. In vitro studies indicate that exposure to high levels of manganese decreases DOPAC levels; manganese excess is associated with Parkinson's-like symptoms. In animal studies, fasting and inhibition of sympathetic nervous system stimulation decreased DOPAC levels. In rats, four days of fasting resulted in decreased DOPAC levels in the stomach and heart, and sympathectomy decreased DOPAC in plasma and muscle. DOPAC levels may be decreased in patients with paroxysmal atrial fibrillation (PAF). Dihydropteridine reductase deficiency (the failure to regenerate tetrahydrobiopterin [BH4], an essential cofactor for tyrosine hydroxylase), decreases plasma DOPAC levels.

Decreased DOPAC may indicate a functional deficiency in monoamine oxidase A (MAO-A) or aldehyde dehydrogenase enzymes. Mutations or single nucleotide polymorphisms (SNPs) in MAO-A genes have been associated with aggression, behavior disorders, alcoholism and attention deficit hyperactivity disorder (ADHD). MAO oxidizes catecholamines and serotonin. MAO also oxidizes amines from the diet and environmental exposures. Amines are widely used in industry and aromatic amines are common in food. Patients with MAO-B deficiency usually have normal plasma DOPAC levels. Animal studies indicate that selenium may improve MAO enzyme function.

MAO and norepinephrine reuptake inhibitors may decrease plasma DOPAC levels. Metyrosine therapy, which decreases the activity of tyrosine hydroxylase (TH), decreases dopamine and may decrease DOPAC levels. TH may also be downregulated by excess catecholamines, oxidative stress, nitrosative stress and thiolation (reactions with sulfur amino acids).

Excess DOPAC may occur in dopamine β-hydroxylase (DβH) deficiency, which results in failure to convert dopamine to norepinephrine, and leads to elevated plasma DOPAC levels. Rat studies indicate that DOPAC levels will increase during acute stressors, but may decrease with prolonged or chronic stress. Increases in L-3,4-dihydroxyphenylalanine (L-DOPA) and dopamine occur after feeding and enter the bloodstream as either DOPAC or dopamine sulfate (animal studies). Administration of reserpine, (which inhibits vesicular uptake of dopamine and increases tyrosine hydroxylase activity) or similar compounds, has been shown to increases plasma DOPAC levels in animals. Forskolin also increases plasma DOPAC levels in animals. Catechol-O-methyl transferase (COMT) enzyme deficiencies increase DOPAC and decrease 3-methoxytyramine (3-MT) levels.

Synthesis and Metabolism:

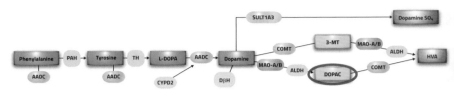

Tyrosine hydroxylase (TH) converts the precursor amino acid tyrosine into L-DOPA. Tyrosine hydroxylase is located in dopamine and norepinephrine neurons in various brain areas. In the periphery, TH is found in the adrenal medulla and in sympathetic ganglia (nerve clusters). Animal studies indicate that selenium deficient diets increase the activity of tyrosine hydroxylase two-fold. Selenium deficiency also decreased the expression of glutathione peroxidase and glutathione reductase; decreased expression of these enzymes may increase intracellular oxidative stress. TH enzyme function may be downregulated by oxidative stress, nitrosative stress and thiolation (reactions with sulfur amino acids). Single nucleotide polymorphisms (SNPs) in the genes coding for tyrosine hydroxylase have been associated with altered stress responses, blood pressure, heart rate and norepinephrine secretion.

L-DOPA is converted to dopamine by DβH; the enzyme requires copper and ascorbate (Vitamin C) cofactors. Dopamine is deaminated and dehydrogenated to form (DOPAC) by monoamine oxidase A (MAOA) and aldehyde dehydrogenase (ALDH). DOPAC is then converted into homovanillic acid (HVA) by catechol-O-methyltransferase (COMT). Deficiency in COMT may elevate DOPAC levels and decrease 3-methoxytyramine (3-MT) levels. COMT requires S-adenosylmethionine (SAM) and a magnesium cofactor. Pre-synaptic uptake and metabolism of dopamine give rise to 3,4-Dihydroxyphenylacetic acid (DOPAC), a different metabolite. Post-synaptic uptake and metabolism produced both DOPAC and 3-MT.

Deficiency in either MAOA or ALDH may result in DOPAC deficiency. Enzyme deficiencies may be inherited or acquired from nutritional deficiency or toxicant exposure. Mutations or single nucleotide polymorphisms (SNPs) in MAOA genes have been associated with aggression, behavior disorders, alcoholism and attention deficit hyperactivity disorder (ADHD). ALDH enzymes have multiple isoforms and three different functional classes; they require a magnesium cofactor. In vitro studies indicate that mitochondrial ALDH2 contributes to neurotransmitter metabolism. Mutations that decrease ALDH2 are common in Asian populations and may severely limit ALDH function. Symptoms of ALDH deficiency include erythema (flushing) of the skin after alcohol consumption, and may include additional symptoms of nausea, headache or physical discomfort. MAOA or ALDH defects may decrease DOPAC and increases 3-MT.

Plasma DOPAC levels are higher that cerebrospinal fluid levels. Experimental evidence indicates that most plasma DOPAC originates in the peripheral nervous system. Animal studies indicate that plasma DOPAC may be partially derived from metabolism of dopamine in noradrenergic (norepinephrine) nerves and that some plasma DOPAC may originate from sympathetic nerves. Plasma DOPAC is also formed from metabolism of dopamine in non-neuronal cells of the gastrointestinal tract. Food ingestion increases plasma DOPAC levels, although the exact effects of diet remain unknown.

Consider:

- Copper levels (**RBC Elements**)

- Magnesium levels (**RBC Elements**)

- Manganese levels (**RBC Elements**)

- Selenium levels (**RBC Elements**)

- MAOA or COMT SNPs (**DNA Methylation Pathway**)

- Methionine metabolism and methylation pathways (**Plasma Methylation Profile, DNA Methylation Pathway**)

- Glutathione status (**Glutathione; erythrocytes**)

- Oxidative stress (**DNA Oxidative Damage Assay/8-OHdG**)

References:

Castaño, A; Ayala, A; Rodriguez-Gomez, J A; de la Cruz, C P; Revilla, E et al. (1995) Increase in dopamine turnover and tyrosine hydroxylase enzyme in hippocampus of rats fed on low selenium diet.
Journal of neuroscience research vol. 42 (5) p. 684-91

Desai, Vishal; Kaler, Stephen G (2008)
Role of copper in human neurological disorders
Am J Clin Nutr vol. 88 (3) p. 855S-858

Eldrup, Ebbe; Richter, Erik A. (2000)
DOPA, dopamine, and DOPAC concentrations in the rat gastrointestinal tract decrease during fasting

Am J Physiol Endocrinol Metab vol. 279 (4) p. E815-822

Eldrup, Ebbe (2004) Significance and origin of DOPA, DOPAC, and dopamine-sulphate in plasma, tissues and cerebrospinal fluid.
Danish Medical Bulletin - No. 1. February 2004. Vol. 51 Pages 34-62.

Goldstein, David S.; Eisenhofer, Graeme; Kopin, Irwin J. (2003)
Sources and Significance of Plasma Levels of Catechols and Their Metabolites in Humans
J. Pharmacol. Exp. Ther. vol. 305 (3) p. 800-811

Rooke, N; Li, D J; Li, J; Keung, W M (2000) The mitochondrial monoamine oxidase-aldehyde dehydrogenase pathway: a potential site of action of daidzin.
Journal of medicinal chemistry vol. 43 (22) p. 4169-79

Sistrunk, Shannon C; Ross, Matthew K; Filipov, Nikolay M (2007)
Direct effects of manganese compounds on dopamine and its metabolite Dopac: an in vitro study.
Environmental toxicology and pharmacology vol. 23 (3) p. 286-96

Wallace, Lane J; Traeger, Jessica S (2012)
Dopac distribution and regulation in striatal dopaminergic varicosities and extracellular space.
Synapse (New York, N.Y.) vol. 66 (2) p. 160-73

Zhou, Wenbo; Gallagher, Amy; Hong, Dong-Pyo; Long, Chunmei; Fink, Anthony L et al. (2009)
At low concentrations, 3,4-dihydroxyphenylacetic acid (DOPAC) binds non-covalently to alpha-synuclein and prevents its fibrillation.
Journal of molecular biology vol. 388 (3) p. 597-610

3-Methoxytyramine (3-MT)

3-Methoxytyramine is the primary extracellular metabolite of Dopamine released from neurons. In mice, 3-MT has been shown to induce behavior changes by binding the trace amine associated receptor 1 (TAAR1). Experimental effects of 3-Methoxytyramine include 3-MT-induced tremor, repetitive behaviors and changes in activity levels (animal studies).

Effects:

Decreased levels of 3-MT may downregulate norepinephrine metabolism, as animal studies indicate that 3-Methoxytyramine accelerates norepinephrine metabolism. Experimental inhibition of catechol-O-methyltransferase (COMT) reduces levels of 3-Methoxytyramine. Metyrosine therapy decreases the activity of tyrosine hydroxylase (TH) and will decrease dopamine levels, which may reduce 3-MT levels. TH function may also be downregulated by high levels of catecholamines, oxidative stress, nitrosative stress and thiolation (reactions with sulfur amino acids).

Excess levels of 3-MT may accelerate norepinephrine metabolism. Animal studies indicate that 3-Methoxytyramine levels may increase during acute stressors, but may habituate to repeated stressors within 10 days. The herbicide Paraquat has been shown to increase 3-MT levels in rats. Deficiency or inhibition of monoamine oxidase (MAO) may elevate 3-MT levels. MAO may be inhibited by cigarette smoke.

Elevations of 3-MT have been associated with a variety of brain and carcinoid tumors. Elevated 3-MT levels may occur in Dopamine-secreting pheochromocytomas, and in paragangliomas. Increases in 3-MT characterized 70% of pheochromocytoma patients with SDHB and SDHD mutations. In some paraganglioma cases, only 3-methoxytyramine is elevated. Plasma levels should always be used to confirm results if catecholamine-producing tumors are suspected. Genetic testing should be considered in all patients with paraganglioma, for as many as 50% of paragangliomas are hereditary.

Synthesis and Metabolism:

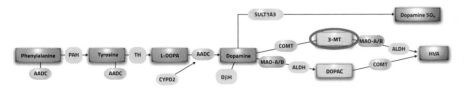

Tyrosine hydroxylase (TH) converts the precursor amino acid tyrosine into L-DOPA. Tyrosine hydroxylase is located in dopamine and norepinephrine neurons in various brain areas. In the periphery, TH is found in the adrenal medulla and in sympathetic ganglia (nerve clusters). Animal studies indicate that selenium deficient diets increase the activity of tyrosine hydroxylase two-fold. Selenium deficiency also decreased the expression of glutathione peroxidase and glutathione reductase; decreased expression of these enzymes may increase intracellular oxidative stress. TH enzyme function may be down regulated by oxidative stress, nitrosative stress and thiolation (reactions with sulfur amino acids). Single nucleotide polymorphisms (SNPs) in the genes coding for tyrosine hydroxylase have been associated with altered stress responses, blood pressure, heart rate and norepinephrine secretion.

L-DOPA is converted to dopamine by amino acid decarboxylase (AADC); the enzyme requires copper and ascorbate (Vitamin C) cofactors. Once released, dopamine is methylated by catechol-O-methyltransferase (COMT). COMT uses S-adenosyl-methionine (SAM) and a magnesium cofactor to degrade dopamine into 3-MT. 3-Methoxytyramine is then further metabolized by monoamine oxidase A (MAO-A) and aldehyde dehydrogenase (ALDH) to homovanillic acid (HVA). Pre-synaptic uptake and metabolism of dopamine give rise to 3,4-Dihydroxyphenylacetic acid (DOPAC), a different metabolite. Post-synaptic uptake and metabolism produced both DOPAC and 3-MT.

Receptors:

3-Methoxytyramine binds with high affinity to alpha-2A adrenergic receptors, and with moderate affinity to alpha-2c1, D_1 and D_2 receptors. The binding of a catechaolamine to an adrenergic receptor usually stimulates the sympathetic nervous system. Experimental inhibition of COMT reduces levels of 3-Methoxytyramine. As COMT is the rate-limiting enzyme, SNPs or mutations that affect COMT enzyme functions may affect levels of 3-Methoxytyramine. The inhibition of monoamine oxidase A (MAO-A) may elevate both 3-MT and normetanephrine levels.

Consider:

- Essential precursor Amino Acid status (**Plasma** or **Urine Amino Acids**)
- Magnesium status
- Selenium status
- MAOA or COMT SNPs (**DNA Methylation Pathway**)
- Methionine metabolism and methylation pathways (**Plasma Methylation Profile, DNA Methylation Pathway**)

References:

Alachkar, Amal; Brotchie, Jonathan M.; Jones, Owen T. (2010) Binding of dopamine and 3-methoxytyramine as l-DOPA metabolites to human 2-adrenergic and dopaminergic receptors *Neuroscience Research* vol. 67 (3) p. 245-249

Antkiewicz-Michaluk, Lucyna; Ossowska, Krystyna; Roma ska, Irena; Michaluk, Jerzy; Vetulani, Jerzy (2008) 3-Methoxytyramine, an extraneuronal dopamine metabolite plays a physiological role in the brain as an inhibitory regulator of catecholaminergic activity *European Journal of Pharmacology* vol. 599 (1) p. 32-35

Booij, L; Van der Does, A J W; Riedel, W J (2003) Monoamine depletion in psychiatric and healthy populations: review *Molecular Psychiatry* (2003) 8, 951–973. doi:10.1038/sj.mp.4001423

Cabib, S.; Puglisi-Allegra, S. (1996) Different effects of repeated stressful experiences on mesocortical and mesolimbic dopamine metabolism *Neuroscience* vol. 73 (2) p. 375-380

Eisenhofer, Graeme; Lenders, Jacques W.M.; Timmers, Henri; Mannelli, Massimo; Grebe, Stefan K. et al. (2011) Measurements of Plasma Methoxytyramine, Normetanephrine, and Metanephrine as Discriminators of Different Hereditary Forms of Pheochromocytoma *Clin. Chem.* vol. 57 (3) p. 411-420

Ossowska, Krystyna; Wardas, Jadwiga; Kuter, Katarzyna; Nowak, Przemysław; Dabrowska, Joanna et al. Influence of paraquat on dopaminergic transporter in the rat brain. *Pharmacological reports : PR* vol. 57 (3) p. 330-5

Sotnikova TD, Beaulieu J-M, Espinoza S, Masri B, Zhang X, et al. (2010) The Dopamine Metabolite 3-Methoxytyramine Is a Neuromodulator. PLoS ONE 5(10): e13452. doi:10.1371/journal.pone.0013452

Young, William F (2006) Paragangliomas: clinical overview. *Annals of the New York Academy of Sciences* vol. 1073 p. 21-9

Norepinephrine

Norepinephrine is secreted by the adrenal gland. Norepinephrine is the primary neurotransmitter for post-ganglionic sympathetic adrenergic nerves (that synapse in target cells). The norephinephrine signaling system regulates the endocrine and autonomic nervous systems. It is the principal neurotransmitter in sympathetic nerve endings. The sympatho-adrenal system plays an important role in the regulation of blood pressure, glucose, sodium concentrations and other physiological and metabolic processes. Norepinephrine binds to adrenergic receptors; the binding of norepinephrine to the receptors primarily stimulates the sympathetic nervous system. Norepinephrine levels may help regulate attention, cognition and sleep. Research indicates that norepinephrine signaling may contribute to:

- Maintaining focus and attention (vigilance)

- Filter weak stimuli and enhance moderate stimuli, and enhance responses to strong stimuli (stimuli are detectable changes in internal or external environment)

- Information processing and executive functions (reasoning, learning, problem-solving)

- Memory storage and retrieval (particularly memories associated with strong emotion)

- "Fight or flight" stress responses

Disregulation of norepinephrine signaling may contribute to mood and bipolar disorders. Evidence indicates that, in the central nervous system (CNS) norepinephrine metabolites are lower in depressed patients and higher during the manic phase of bipolar patients. Medications that prevent norepinephrine reuptake or inhibit norepinephrine metabolism have been shown to improve depressive symptoms.

Effects:

Decreased norepinephrine may be associated with rare, inherited conditions such as dopamine beta-hydroxylase (DβH) enzyme deficiency and Menkes disease. Elevated dopamine (and metabolites) and low norepinephrine levels may occur due to DβH enzyme dysfunctions. Multiple single nucleotide polymorphisms (SNPs) have been identified in the genes coding for DβH and are being evaluated for associations in attention, behavior, psychiatric and neuro-degenerative disorders. Symptoms of norepinephrine insufficiency, which may be seen in $D\beta H$ enzyme deficiencies, may include:

- Cardiovascular disease
- Severe orthostatic hypotension
- Droopy eyelids
- Stuffy nose
- Reduced muscle tone
- Recurring low blood sugar
- Adrenaline deficiency
- Ejaculation problems
- Exercise intolerance

Stimulation of alpha-2-adrenoreceptors (alpha-2 agonist medication) decreases sympathetic nerve outflow and norepinephrine levels. Surgical sympathectomies or medical conditions that disrupt autonomic nerve functions may also decrease norepinephrine levels. Alpha- and beta-blocker medications may decrease norepinephrine levels. Metyrosine therapy decreases levels of the precursor neurotransmitter dopamine and may reduce norepinephrine and normetanephrine levels. Medications that may reduce norepinephrine and normetanephrine levels include anti-hypertensives (blood pressure), serotonin reuptake inhibitors, heart medications and lithium.

Excess urinary norepinephrine (and cortisol) levels have been associated with anxiety. The Heart and Soul Study (2005) associated elevated urinary norepinephrine with depressive symptoms in patients with cardiac disease. Symptoms of excess norepinephrine may include:

- Hypertension

- Palpitations or arrhythmia
- Anxiety or nervousness
- Nausea and vomiting
- Abdominal pain
- Chest pain
- Irritability
- Pallor
- Sweating
- Weight loss
- Hand tremor
- Insomnia

Impaired re-uptake of norepinephrine by neurons has been associated with congestive heart failure (CHF). Postural tachycardia syndrome (POTS), an orthostatic tachycardia primarily affecting women, is associated with elevated plasma norepinephrine levels; a 24-hour urine catecholamines assessment may be used as an alternative. Mutations in the cell membrane norepinephrine transporters (NET) may alter function and increase norepinephrine levels. Patients with NET mutations may have excessive increases in heart rate and plasma norepinephrine levels when standing. Altered NET function has been associated with attention deficit hyperactivity disorder (ADHD). Norepinephrine re-uptake inhibitor (NRI) and some selective serotonin reuptake inhibitor (SSRI) medications may elevate norepinephrine levels by inhibiting NET function. The down-regulation of alpha-2-adrenoceptors may increase sympathetic nerve outflow and norepinephrine levels. Medications, such as beta-adrenoreceptor agonists, may increase norepinephrine release into plasma.

Phenylethanolamine N-methyltransferase (PNMT) catalyzes the synthesis of epinephrine from norepinephrine. PNMT requires S-adenosyl methionine (SAM) as a cofactor. Elevated norepinephrine and low epinephrine levels may occur if PNMT enzyme function is deficient. Serious illness, physical activity or stress may cause temporary increases in norepinephrine and other catecholamines. Pheochromocytoma tumors may secrete norepinephrine.

Elevations in norepinephrine and blood pressure may result in severe throbbing headaches. Tyramine and other sympathomimetic amines, promote the release of norepinephrine from nerve endings. If monoamine oxidase a (MAO-A) is inhibited by medication or if enzyme function is deficient, tyramine is able to reach the sympathetic nerve terminals, and paroxysmal hypertension may result from release of vesicular norepinephrine. Short-term fasting (four days) has been shown to elevate plasma norepinephrine levels, as has the ingestion of glucose.

Synthesis and Metabolism:

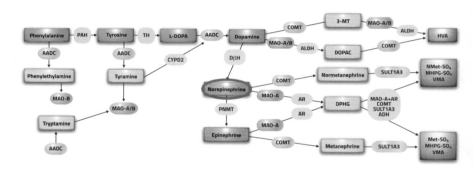

Synthesis begins with the conversion of tyrosine to 3,4-dihydroxyphenylalanine (L-DOPA) by the enzyme tyrosine-3-hydrolase (TH). Lack of nutrient cofactors may decrease TH function; TH requires tetrahydrobiopterin (BH4) and iron for normal function. Tyrosine hydroxylase is located in dopamine and norepinephrine neurons in various brain areas. In the periphery, TH is found in the adrenal medulla and in sympathetic ganglia (nerve clusters). Animal studies indicate that selenium deficient diets increase the activity of tyrosine hydroxylase two-fold. Selenium deficiency also decreased the expression of glutathione

peroxidase and glutathione reductase; decreased expression of these enzymes may increase intracellular oxidative stress. TH enzyme function may be downregulated by oxidative stress, nitrosative stress and thiolation (reactions with sulfur amino acids). Single nucleotide polymorphisms (SNPs) in the genes coding for tyrosine hydroxylase have been associated with altered stress responses, blood pressure, heart rate and norepinephrine secretion.

Dopamine is an intermediate metabolite in the synthesis of norepinephrine; L-DOPA is converted to dopamine by aromatic amino acid decarboxylase (AADC), using pyridoxal phosphate (B6). Dopamine beta-hydroxylase (DβH) then converts dopamine to norepinephrine. DβH requires a copper cofactor, and abnormal copper transport may decrease DβH activity. Norepinephrine and other catecholamines are sequestered in vesicles by vesicular monoamine transporters (VMAT) until released. The function of VMAT may also influence norepinephrine levels; plasma norepinephrine levels are determined mainly by release from intracellular vesicles. Reuptake occurs through the norepinephrine transporter (NET) in the cell membrane. Sulfotransferase (SULT) enzymes are not found in neurons. SULT1A3 catabolizes normetanephrine and its activity may decrease in liver disease. SULT activity has been down-regulated in vitro by coffee compounds, green tea polyphenols, quercitin and resveratrol. SULT enzymes also conjugate a variety of xenobiotic chemicals that may be inhaled or ingested during environmental exposures. Some SULT enzymes are sensitive to regulation by hormones, others conjugate hormones. Research continues in this area.

Although norepinephrine and epinephrine are primarily metabolized in the same cells where they are synthesized, catecholamine metabolism varies greatly between body organs. Sympathetic nerves contain monoamine oxidase (MAO) but not catechol-O-methyltransferase (COMT). Adrenal cells contain both MAO and COMT enzymes. COMT uses S-adenosyl-methionine (SAM) and a magnesium cofactor; selenium may improve MAO function. Normetanephrine is a norepinephrine metabolite of COMT, and is exclusively an extra-neuronal metabolite. Contrary

to usual depictions of catecholamine metabolism, vanillylmandelic acid (VMA) is primarily produced by oxidation of norepinephrine metabolite 3-methoxy-4-hydroxyphenylglycol (MHPG), and metabolized by alcohol and aldehyde dehydrogenases. The presence of a beta-hydroxyl group on norepinephrine, epinephrine and their metabolites favors reduction by aldehyde or aldose reductases. Metabolites measured in the mesenteric organs indicate that about half of all norepinephrine is produced in the gastrointestinal tract, pancreas, and spleen. Most of the norepinephrine produced by mesenteric organs is removed by the from portal vein blood by the liver and converted to VMA for excretion. Uptake of circulating catecholamines by the liver and kidney, while important for the clearance of catecholamines, contributes less than 25% of the total metabolism of catecholamines.

Receptors

Adrenergic receptors bind catecholamine neurotransmitters such as norepinephrine and epinephrine. If signaled by the CNS, preganglionic nerves using acetylcholine neurotransmitters will stimulate postganglionic nerves to secrete norepinephrine into target receptor synapses in cells and tissues. The binding of norepinephrine to the receptors primarily stimulates the sympathetic nervous system. Norepinephrine concentrations in the target receptor's synapse is regulated by the CNS and pre-ganglionic neurons.

Alpha adrenergic receptors affect vasoconstriction and gastrointestinal motility. There are multiple adrenergic receptor subtypes; each is encoded separately in the DNA. Alpha receptors stimulate the production of second messenger molecule inositol 1,4,5-trisphosphate (IP3), which regulates calcium-mediated functions.

- alpha1 receptors – increase smooth muscle contraction; they contribute to the regulation of sodium re-absorption in the kidney and glucose metabolism in adipose tissue and astroglia (astrocytes) in the nervous system. The receptors modulate cellular calcium flux and cellular signaling via secondary messenger molecules. $\alpha 1$ receptors are considered post-synaptic and stimulatory in the CNS. Recent evidence indicates that the receptors may contribute to CNS locomotor functions. Over-expression of $\alpha 1B$ receptors in a mouse model results in symptoms of Parkisnon's disease, autonomic failure and multiple system atrophy.

- alpha2 receptors – are found on both pre-a and post-synaptic cells and inhibit the release of norepinephrine, acetylcholine and insulin. The downregulation of $\alpha 12$-adrenoceptors may increase sympathetic nerve outflow and norepinephrine levels. The amino acid leucine has been shown to downregulate $\alpha 12$ adrenergic receptor expression. Down-regulation of $\alpha 12$ adrenoceptors has been associated with inflammatory bowel disease in animal models. In vitro studies suggest that tumor necrosis factor alpha (TNF-α) and interferon gamma (IFN-γ) may also downregulate alpha-2 adrenoreceptors.

Beta (β) adrenergic receptors signal cells through cAMP, protein kinase A, and phosphorylation of proteins. Thyroid function and T3 levels, may affect norepinephrine signaling in the CNS, and increase β-adrenergic receptor activity.

- beta1 receptors – are primarily found in the heart and kidney. In the heart, stimulation of $\beta 1$ receptors increases heart rate and contractility. In the kidney, receptor stimulation results in the release of rennin.

- beta2 receptors – are found in a variety of involuntary muscles, such as the bladder detrusor muscle, the eye cilliary muscle and vascular smooth muscles. Stimulation of the receptor relaxes these muscles and decreases gastrointestinal motility. In the liver, $\beta 2$ stimulation increases glucose activation and lipolysis (fat breakdown).

- beta3 receptors – stimulation of these receptors promotes lipolysis.

Single nucleotide polymorphisms (SNPs) in the DNA coding for adrenergic receptors may affect their structure and function. A variety of medications target specific types of adrenergic receptors and may influence norepinephrine levels and signaling.

Consider:

Tyrosine on an empty stomach may improve transport across BBB; may be contraindicated in hypertension; may induce anxiety in some patients.

Further evaluations:

- Essential precursor Amino Acid status (**Plasma** or **Urine Amino Acids**)

- Copper status (**RBC Elements**)

- Iron status (**RBC Elements**)

- Magnesium levels (**RBC elements**)

- Selenium status (**RBC Elements**)

- Glutathione status (Glutathione; erythrocytes)
- Oxidative stress (DNA Oxidative Damage Assay/8-OHdG)
- Methionine metabolism and methylation pathways (Plasma Methylation Profile, DNA Methylation Pathway)

References:

Bauer, M.; Heinz, A.; Whybrow, P.C.(2002)
Thyroid hormones, serotonin and mood: of synergy and significance in the adult brain
Nature Publishing Group vol. 7 (2)

Castaño, A; Ayala, A; Rodriguez-Gomez, J A; de la Cruz, C P; Revilla, E et al. (1995)
Increase in dopamine turnover and tyrosine hydroxylase enzyme in hippocampus of rats fed on low selenium diet.
Journal of neuroscience research vol. 42 (5) p. 684-91

Davis, Kenneth L, et al.,, Editors
Neuropsychopharmacology: The Fifth Generation of Progress
Lippincott, Williams, & Wilkins, Philadelphia, Pennsylvania, 2002

Dong, Jun-hong; Chen, Xin; Cui, Min; Yu, Xiao; Pang, Qi et al. (2012)
2-adrenergic receptor and astrocyte glucose metabolism.
Journal of molecular neuroscience : MN vol. 48 (2) p. 456-63

Eisenhofer, Graeme; Kopin, Irwin J.; Goldstein, David S. (2004)
Catecholamine Metabolism: A Contemporary View with Implications for Physiology and Medicine
Pharmacol. Rev. vol. 56 (3) p. 331-349

Goldstein, David S.; Eisenhofer, Graeme; Kopin, Irwin J. (2003)

Sources and Significance of Plasma Levels of Catechols and Their Metabolites in Humans
J. Pharmacol. Exp. Ther. vol. 305 (3) p. 800-811

Guzmán, Flavio, MD.
University of Mendoza, Argentina
http://pharmacologycorner.com/
Accessed 04 December 2014

Kodirov, Sodikdjon A. (2012)
The Amygdala - A Discrete Multitasking Manager
InTech. ISBN 978-953-51-0908-2

Piascik, Michael T.; Perez, Dianne M. (2001)
alpha 1-Adrenergic Receptors: New Insights and Directions
J. Pharmacol. Exp. Ther. vol. 298 (2) p. 403-410

Otte, Christian; Neylan, Thomas C.; Pipkin, Sharon S.; Browner, Warren S.; Whooley, Mary A. (2005)
Depressive Symptoms and 24-Hour Urinary Norepinephrine Excretion Levels in Patients With Coronary Disease: Findings From the Heart and Soul Study
American Journal of Psychiatry vol. 162 (11) p. 2139-2145

Owens, Michael J; Krulewicz, Stan; Simon, Jeffrey S; Sheehan, David V; Thase, Michael E et al. (2008)
Estimates of Serotonin and Norepinephrine Transporter Inhibition in Depressed Patients Treated with Paroxetine or Venlafaxine
American College of Neuropsychopharmacology vol. 33 (13) p. 3201-3212

Soliman,Kamal; Sturman,Steve; Sarkar,Prabodh K.; Michael,Atef (2010)
Postural orthostatic tachycardia syndrome (POTS): a diagnostic dilemma.
February 2010 Volume 17, Issue 1 Br J Cardiol 2010;17:36-9

Zauner, Christian; Schneeweiss, Bruno; Kranz, Alexander; Madl, Christian; Ratheiser, Klaus et al. (2000) Resting energy expenditure in short-term starvation is increased as a result of an increase in serum norepinephrine *Am J Clin Nutr* vol. 71 (6) p. 1511-1515

Normetanephrine

Normetanephrine is a metabolite of norepinephrine. The adrenal glands are the single largest source of normetanephrine. Between 25-40% of circulating normetanephrine is derived from catecholamine metabolism from the adrenal medulla. Both the catecholamines and their metabolites are excreted in the urine. In the normal population, plasma metanephrine and normetanephrine levels are low. Normetanephrine inhibits low affinity, high capacity biogenic amine transporters such as organic cation transporters (OCTs) and the plasma membrane monoamine transporter (PMAT). These nonspecific transporters are highly expressed in the brain, and participate in the clearance of monoamine neurotransmitters from synapses in to prevent neurotransmitter excess. Clinically, normetanephrine provides an index of norepinephrine released due to sympathetic nerve activity.

Effects:

Decreased levels of normetanephrine may occur when norepinephrine levels decrease. Low normetanephrine levels may occur if catechol-O-methyltransferase (COMT) function is deficient. Pure autonomic failure is associated with low levels of norepinephrine and normetanephrine. Rare, inherited conditions such as dopamine beta-hydroxylase (DβH) deficiency and Menkes disease may also decrease norepineph-

rine and normetanephrine levels. DβH requires a copper cofactor. Multiple single nucleotide polymorphisms (SNPs) have been identified in the genes coding for DβH and are being evaluated for associations in attention, behavior, psychiatric and neurodegenerative disorders Symptoms of norepinephrine insufficiency, which may be seen in DβH enzyme deficiencies, may include:

- Cardiovascular disease
- Severe orthostatic hypotension
- Droopy eyelids
- Stuffy nose
- Reduced muscle tone
- Recurring low blood sugar
- Adrenaline deficiency
- Ejaculation problems

  Exercise intolerance

Metyrosine therapy decreases levels of the precursor neurotransmitter dopamine and may reduce norepinephrine and normetanephrine levels Medications that may reduce norepinephrine and normetanephrine levels include anti-hypertensives (blood pressure), serotonin reuptake inhibitors heart medications and lithium.

Excess normetanephrine may occur if sulfotransferase (SULT) or Phenylethanolamine N-methyltransferase (PNMT) enzyme function is deficient. PNMT catalyzes the synthesis of epinephrine from norepinephrine. PNMT requires S-adenosyl methionine (SAM) as a cofactor. Elevated norepinephrine and low epinephrine levels may occur if PNMT enzyme function is deficient. Most catecholamines are metabolized in the cells that produce them; normetanephrine levels may elevate when norepinephrine levels elevate. Decreased function of sulfotransferase (SULT) enzymes may elevate normetanephrine and metanephrine levels. SULTs are not found in neurons. SULT activity has been down-regulated in vitro by coffee compounds, green tea polyphenols, quercitin and resveratrol. SULT enzymes also conjugate a variety of xenobiotic chemicals that may be inhaled or ingested during environmental exposures. SULT1A3 converts norepinephrine to normetanephrine and its activity is decreased in liver disease.

Studies indicate that hypertensive males with obstructive sleep apnea have higher urinary normetanephrine levels. Norepinephrine and normetanephrine may elevate when catecholamine-secreting tumors are present. See Adrenal and paraganglia tumors for more information. Excess norepinephrine and normetanephrine symptoms may include:

- Hypertension
- Palpitations or arrhythmia
- Anxiety or nervousness
- Nausea and vomiting
- Abdominal pain
- Chest pain
- Irritability
- Pallor
- Sweating
- Weight loss
- Hand tremor
- Insomnia

Normetanephrine is usually present in the urine in small fluctuating amounts and may be increased during and shortly after stress exposures. Medications that inhibit the reuptake of norepinephrine or serotonin may also elevate normetanephrine levels.

Synthesis and Metabolism:

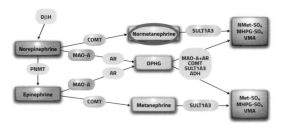

Once released, norepinephrine is metabolized to normetanephrine. Adrenomedullary chromaffin cells possess catechol-O-methyltransferase (COMT) and the metabolism 25-40% of norepinephrine in the adrenal medulla occurs before the neurotransmitter is released. COMT requires a magnesium cofactor. COMT is not found in sympathetic nerves, but monoamine oxidase A (MAO-A) is. Contrary to usual depictions of catecholamine metabolism, vanillylmandelic acid (VMA) is primarily produced by oxidation of norepinephrine metabolite 3-methoxy-4-hydroxyphenylglycol (MHPG), and metabolized by alcohol and aldehyde dehydrogenases. The presence of a beta-hydroxyl group on norepinephrine, epinephrine and their metabolites favors reduction by aldehyde or aldose reductases. The deamination of norepinephrine and epinephrine by monoamine oxidase A (MAO-A) and the subsequent formation of VMA have a minimal effect on catecholamine catabolism in neurons.

Evidence indicates that sulfate-conjugated normetanephrine is instead formed primarily in gastrointestinal tissue. SULT activity has been down-regulated in vitro by coffee compounds, green tea polyphenols, quercitin and resveratrol. SULT enzymes also conjugate a variety of xenobiotic chemicals that may be inhaled or ingested during environmental exposures. SULT1A3 converts norepinephrine to normetanephrine and its activity may decrease in liver disease.

In urinary assays, free normetanephrines represent a small proportion (<3%) of the total measured normetanephrines. Doctor's Data measures total normetanephrines, which is the medical convention.

Consider:

- Copper status (**RBC Elements**)
- Magnesium status (**RBC Elements**)
- Status of neurotransmitter precursor Phenylalanine (**Amino Acids**)
- Glutathione status (**Glutathione; erythrocytes**)
- MAOA or COMT SNPs (**DNA Methylation Pathway**)
- Methionine metabolism and methylation pathways (**Plasma Methylation Profile, DNA Methylation Pathway**)
- Oxidative stress/8OH-dG (**DNA Oxidative Damage Assay**)

References:

American Association for Clinical Chemistry (2010)
Urine Metanephrines
http://labtestsonline.org/understanding/ analytes/urine-metanephrine/tab/sample/
accessed 04 Aug 2014

Coughtrie, Michael W. H.; Johnston, Laura E. (2001)
Interactions between Dietary Chemicals and Human Sulfotransferases{---}Molecular Mechanisms and Clinical Significance
Drug Metab. Dispos. vol. 29 (4) p. 522-528

Daubner, S Colette; Le, Tiffany; Wang, Shanzhi (2011)
Tyrosine hydroxylase and regulation of dopamine synthesis.
Archives of biochemistry and biophysics vol. 508 (1) p. 1-12

Eisenhofer, Graeme; Lenders, Jacques W.M.; Timmers, Henri; Mannelli, Massimo; Grebe, Stefan K. et al. (2011)
Measurements of Plasma Methoxytyramine, Normetanephrine, and Metanephrine as Discriminators of Different Hereditary Forms of Pheochromocytoma
Clin. Chem. vol. 57 (3) p. 411-420

Eisenhofer, Graeme; Kopin, Irwin J.; Goldstein, David S. (2004)
Catecholamine Metabolism: A Contemporary View with Implications for Physiology and Medicine
Pharmacol. Rev. vol. 56 (3) p. 331-349

Eisenhofer, Graeme (2001)
Free or Total Metanephrines for Diagnosis of Pheochromocytoma: What Is the Difference?
Clin. Chem. vol. 47 (6) p. 988-989

Elmasry, A.; Lindberg, E.; Hedner, J.; Janson, C.; Boman, G. (2002)
Obstructive sleep apnoea and urine catecholamines in hypertensive males: a population-based study
Eur. Respir. J. vol. 19 (3) p. 511-517

Goldstein, David S (2010)
Catecholamines 101.
Clinical autonomic research : official journal of the Clinical Autonomic Research Society vol. 20 (6) p. 331-52

Jong, Wilhelmina H. A. de; Eisenhofer, Graeme; Post, Wendy J.; Muskiet, Frits A. J.; Vries, Elisabeth G. E. de et al. (2013)
Dietary Influences on Plasma and Urinary Metanephrines: Implications for Diagnosis of Catecholamine-Producing Tumors
Endocrine Society

Oeltmann, Timothy; Carson, Robert; Shannon, John R.; Ketch, Terry; Robertson, David (2004)
Assessment of O-methylated catecholamine levels in plasma and urine for diagnosis of autonomic disorders
Autonomic Neuroscience vol. 116 (1) p. 1-10

Vialou, V.; Balasse, L.; Dumas, S.; Giros, B.; Gautron, S. (2007)
Neurochemical characterization of pathways expressing plasma membrane mono-amine transporter in the rat brain
Neuroscience vol. 144 (2) p. 616-622

Yalcin, Emine B.; More, Vijay; Neira, Karissa L.; Lu, Zhenqiang James; Cherrington, Nathan J. et al. (2013)
Downregulation of Sulfotransferase Expression and Activity in Diseased Human Livers
Drug Metab. Dispos. vol. 41 (9) p. 1642-1650

Epinephrine

Small amounts of epinephrine are constantly secreted to maintain normal blood pressure and metabolic functions. Evidence is accumulating that epinephrine has neurotransmitter-like functions in the CNS that may affect the regulation of blood pressure, respiration, and pituitary hormone secretion.

Clinically, plasma epinephrine levels have been shown to reflect central nervous system (CNS) neural outflow to the adrenal medulla. Virtually all circulating epinephrine originates from the adrenal medulla.

Effects:

Decreased epinephrine levels may occur in conditions such as Addison's disease, diabetic nephropathy, congenital 21-hydroxylase deficiency and Autonomic Failure syndromes. Alpha- and beta-blocker medications may reduce the effects of epinephrine, but are not documented to reduce systemic epinephrine levels. Metyrosine therapy decreases levels of the precursor neurotransmitters dopamine and norepinephrine, and may reduce epinephrine levels.

Excess or elevated levels of epinephrine may be secreted during acute stress (fight or flight response). Short-term stress-response elevations increase heart rate, blood pressure, muscle strength and blood glucose levels, and decrease insulin levels, parasympathetic and digestive functions. Virtually all circulating epinephrine present during the "stress response" originates from the adrenal medulla. Epinephrine elevations have been documented in extreme exercise, panic attacks and some cases of essential hypertension. Plasma epinephrine levels have been shown to elevate in response to global metabolic threats, such as shock (hypoglycemia, hemorrhagic hypotension, asphyxia, circulatory collapse) and also during emotional distress. Serious illness and stress can cause moderate to large temporary increases in catecholamine levels.

Postural tachycardia syndrome (POTS) patients may have elevated plasma epinephrine while at rest. Experimental administration of epinephrine to men decreased thyroid hormone metabolism and free T4 levels, and increased thyroid hormone binding globulin levels. Experimental administration of epinephrine to male Type II diabetics altered the metabolism of glycerol, non-esterified fatty acids and triacylglycerols in adipose tissues. Mild, asymptomatic hypoglycemia may increase epinephrine compared to norepinephrine levels. Elevated epinephrine concentrations may decrease the serum potassium concentrations. Epinephrine:norepinphrine ratios may increase after surgical sympathectomy. Symptoms of elevated epinephrine may include:

- Headaches (severe)
- High blood pressure
- Excess sweating (generalized)
- Racing heart (tachycardia)
- Anxiety or nervousness
- Tremors
- Epigastric pain (lower chest or upper abdomen)
- Nausea or vomiting
- Weight loss
- Heat intolerance

Epinephrine is usually present in the urine in small fluctuating amounts and may be increased during and shortly after stress exposures. Monoamine oxidase inhibitors (MAOIs) may elevate epinephrine and metanephrine levels. Drugs that stimulate nicotinic, angiotensin II, or glucagon receptors may also increase plasma epinephrine levels.

Synthesis and Metabolism:

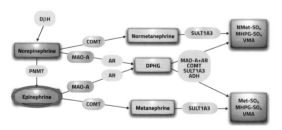

Enephrine is primarily synthesized in the chromaffin cells of the adrenal medulla; small amounts are synthesized in the Central Nervous System (CNS) and the vagus nerve. Epinephrine is derived from norepinephrine. Phenylethanolamine N-methyltransferase (PNMT) methylates norepinephrine to form epinephrine, using S-adenosyl methionine (SAM) as a cofactor. High concentrations of PNMT are found in the adrenal medulla, and PNMT is found in certain areas of the brain and vagus nerve. Individual production and response to epinephrine levels may be influenced in part by genetic polymorphisms (SNPs) in the PNMT enzyme. Animal studies indicate that PNMT activity may be upregulated by excercies, high cortisol levels (such corticosteroid medications) or stress. Epinephrine is stored in vesicles until it is released into the circulation.

Adrenomedullary chromaffin cells possess monoamine oxidase A (MAO-A) and catechol-O-methyl transferase (COMT). Approximately 90% of epinephrine is metabolized before the neurotransmitter is released. COMT equires a magnesium cofactor and -adenosylmethionine. COMT is not ound in sympathetic nerves, but monomine oxidase A (MAO-A) is. Contrary o usual depictions of catecholamine netabolism, vanillylmandelic acid VMA) is primarily produced by the xidation of the epinephrine metabote 3-methoxy-4-hydroxyphenylglycol MHPG), and is metabolized by alcool and aldehyde dehydrogenases. The resence of a beta-hydroxyl group on pinephrine, norepinephrine and their netabolites favors reduction by aldeyde or aldose reductases. Uptake of irculating catecholamines by the liver and kidney, while important for the learance of catacholamines, contributes ess than 25% of the total metabolism of atecholamines. Circulating epinephrine inactivated by cacatechol-O-methtransferase (COMT) in the liver. The learance of catecholamines from the lood requires several passes through ne hepatic circulation.

Sulfotransferase (SULT) enzymes atabolize metanephrine; decreased enyme activity increase metanephrine evels. SULT enzymes are not found n neurons. SULT activity has been own-regulated in vitro by coffee comounds, green tea polyphenols, quercitin nd resveratrol. SULT enzymes also conugate a variety of xenobiotic chemicals nat may be inhaled or ingested during nvironmental exposures.

eceptors

Adrenergic receptors bind catecholmine neurotransmitters such as norepiephrine and epinephrine.

Alpha (α) adrenergic receptors afct vasoconstriction and gastrointestial motility. There are multiple adrenrgic receptor subtypes; each is encoded

separately in the DNA. Alpha receptors stimulate the production of second messenger molecule 1,4,5-trisphosphate (IP3), which regulates calcium-mediated functions. Epinephrine binding to α2-adrenergic receptors constricts arteries in the gut, skin, and kidney.

alpha1 receptors – increase smooth muscle contraction, they contribute the regulation of sodium re-absorption in the kidney and glucose metabolism in adipose tissue and astroglia (astrocytes) in the nervous system. The receptors modulate cellular calcium flux and cellular signaling via secondary messenger molecules. α1 receptors are considered post-synaptic and stimulatory in the CNS. Recent evidence indicates that the receptors may contribute to CNS locomotor functions. Over-expression of α1B receptors in a mouse model results in symptoms of Parkisnon's disease, autonomic failure and multiple system atrophy.

alpha2 receptors – are found on both pre-a and post-synaptic cells and inhibit the release of norepinephrine, acetylcholine and insulin. The downregulation of α-2-adrenoceptors may increase sympathetic nerve outflow and norepinephrine levels.

Beta (β) adrenergic receptors signal cells through cAMP, protein kinase A, and phosphorylation of proteins. The binding of epinephrine to β-adrenergic receptors on liver and adipose cells releases glucose and fatty acids, and relaxes vascular smooth muscle in the gut, skin, and kidney. Thyroid function and T3 levels may increase β-adrenergic receptor activity.

- beta1 receptors – are primarily found in the heart and kidney. In the heart, stimulation of β1 receptors increases heart rate and contractility.

In the kidney, receptor stimulation results in the release of rennin.

- beta2 receptors – are found in a variety of involuntary muscles, such as the bladder detrusor muscle, the eye cilliary muscle and vascular smooth muscles. Stimulation of the receptor relaxes these muscles and decreases gastrointestinal motility. In the liver, $\beta2$ stimulation increases glucose activation and lipolysis (fat breakdown).

- beta3 receptors – stimulation of these receptors promotes lipolysis.

Single nucleotide polymorphisms (SNPs) in the DNA coding for adrenergic receptors may affect their structure and function. A variety of medications target specific types of adrenergic receptors and may influence norepinephrine levels and signaling.

Consider:

- Copper status (**RBC Elements**)

- Magnesium status (**RBC Elements**)

- Status of neurotransmitter precursor Phenylalanine (**Amino Acids**)

- MAOA or COMT SNPs (**DNA Methylation Pathway**)

References:

Bauer, M.; Heinz, A.; Whybrow, P.C.(2002)
Thyroid hormones, serotonin and mood:
of synergy and significance in the adult brain
Nature Publishing Group vol. 7 (2)

Goldstein, David S (2010)
Catecholamines 101.
Clinical autonomic research : official journal of the Clinical Autonomic Research Society vol. 20 (6) p. 331-52

Hays, M T; Solomon, D H (1969)
Effect of epinephrine on the peripheral metabolism of thyroxine.
The Journal of clinical investigation vol. 48 (6 p. 1114-23

Ji, Yuan; Snyder, Eric M.; Fridley, Brooke L.; Salavaggione, Oreste E.; Moon, Irene et al. (2008)
Human phenylethanolamine N-methyltransferase genetic polymorphisms and exercise-induced epinephrine release
Physiol Genomics vol. 33 (3) p. 323-332

Tobin, L; Simonsen, L; Galbo, H; Bülow, J (2012)
Vascular and metabolic effects of adrenaline in adipose tissue in type 2 diabetes.
Nutrition & diabetes vol. 2 p. e46

Wu, Qian; Caine, Joanne M; Thomson, Stuart A; Slavica, Meri; Grunewald, Gary L et al. (2009)
Time-dependent inactivation of human phenylethanolamine N-methyltransferase by 7-isothiocyanatotetrahydroisoquinoline.
Bioorganic & medicinal chemistry letters vol. 19 (4) p. 1071-4

Ziegler, Michael G; Aung, Myo; Kennedy, Brian (1997)
Sources of human urinary epinephrine
International Society of Nephrology vol. 51 (1 p. 324-327

Metanephrine

Metanephrine is a metabolite of epi nephrine. The adrenal glands are the single largest source of metanephrine Approximately 90% of circulating me tanephrine is derived from catechol amine metabolism in the adrenal me dulla. Both the catecholamines and thei metabolites are excreted in the urine In the normal population, plasma me tanephrine and normetanephrine level are low. Clinically, metanephrine level provide an indication of the adrenal me dulla's metabolism of epinephrine prior to its release into circulation.

Effects:

Decreased levels of metanephrine may occur when epinephrine levels decrease. Phenylethanolamine N-methyltransferase (PNMT) deficiency or 21-dehydroxylase deficiency may decrease epinephrine and metanephrine levels. Studies indicate that 21-dehydroxylase deficiency may decrease plasma epinephrine and metanephrine concentrations and urinary epinephrine excretion by 40 to 80%. PNMT deficiency may also elevate norepinephrine levels. Decreased metanephrine levels may occur if catechol-O-methyltransferase (COMT) function is deficient or inhibited in adrenal cells. COMT requires magnesium and S-adenosyl-methionine cofactors.

Pure autonomic failure is associated with low levels of epinephrine and metanephrine. Rare, inherited conditions such as dopamine beta-hydroxylase (DβH) deficiency and Menkes disease may also decrease levels of norepinephrine, the precursor for epinephrine. DβH requires a copper cofactor. There is little literature describing the symptoms of pure epinephrine (and/or metanephrine) deficiency, however, conditions that may be associated with low epinephrine levels include Addison's disease, diabetic nephropathy and autonomic failure syndromes.

Excess metanephrine may occur if sulfotransferase (SULT) enzyme function is deficient. Metanephrines may be elevated in anxiety disorders or bipolar disorders. Physical conditions, including congestive heart failure, porphyria, hyperthyroidism and some autoimmune conditions. Most catecholamines are metabolized in the cells that produce them; metanephrine levels may elevate when epinephrine levels elevate. Studies indicate that hypertensive males with obstructive sleep apnea have higher urinary metanephrine and normetanephrine levels. Epinephrine and metanephrine may elevate when catecholamine-secreting tumors are present. See Adrenal and paraganglia tumors for more information. Excess metanephrine symptoms (excess epinephrine symptoms) may include:

Symptoms of elevated epinephrine may include:

- Headaches (severe)
- High blood pressure
- Excess sweating (generalized)
- Racing heart (tachycardia)
- Anxiety or nervousness
- Tremors
- Epigastric pain (lower chest or upper abdomen)
- Nausea or vomiting
- Weight loss
- Heat intolerance

Epinephrine is usually present in the urine in small fluctuating amounts and may be increased during and shortly after stress exposures. Monoamine oxidase inhibitors may elevate epinephrine and metanephrine levels.

Synthesis and metabolism:

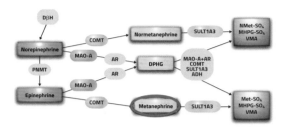

Norepinephrine is converted to epinephrine by phenylethanolamine N-methyltransferase (PNMT). PNMT requires an S-adenosyl methionine (SAM) cofactor. Animal studies indicate that PNMT activity may be upregulated by exercise, high cortisol levels (such corticosteroid medications) or stress. Epinephrine is stored in vesicles until it is released into the circulation.

Metanephrine is produced outside of neurons (extra-neuronally). Adrenomedullary chromaffin cells possess monoamine oxidase A (MAO-A) and catechol-O-methyl transferase (COMT). Approximately 90% of epinephrine is metabolized before the neurotransmitter is released. COMT requires a magnesium cofactor and S-adenosylmethionine. COMT is not found in sympathetic nerves, but monoamine oxidase A (MAO-A) is. Contrary to usual depictions of catecholamine metabolism, vanillylmandelic acid (VMA) is primarily produced by the oxidation of the epinephrine metabolite 3-methoxy-4-hydroxyphenylglycol (MHPG), and is metabolized by alcohol and aldehyde dehydrogenases. The presence of a beta-hydroxyl group on epinephrine, norepinephrine and their metabolites favors reduction by aldehyde or aldose reductases. Uptake of circulating catecholamines by the liver and kidney, while important for the clearance of catacholamines, contributes less than 25% of the total metabolism of catecholamines.

Evidence indicates that sulfate-conjugated normetanephrine is instead formed primarily in gastrointestinal tissue. Sulfotransferase (SULT) enzymes are not found in neurons. SULT activity has been down-regulated *in vitro* by coffee compounds, green tea polyphenols, quercitin and resveratrol. SULT enzymes also conjugate a variety of xenobiotic chemicals that may be inhaled or ingested during environmental exposures. Some SULT enzymes are sensitive to regulation by hormones, others conjugate hormones. SULT1A3 converts epinephrine to metanephrine and its activity may decrease in liver disease, elevating levels of metanephrine and normetanephrine.

In urinary assays, free metanephrines represent a small proportion (<3%) of the total measured normetanephrines. Doctor's Data measures total metanephrines, which is the medical convention.

Consider:

- Copper status (**RBC Elements**)
- Magnesium status (**RBC Elements**)
- Status of neurotransmitter precursor Phenylalanine (**Amino Acids**)

Glutathione status (**Glutathione; erythrocytes**)

- Oxidative stress/8OH-dG (**DNA Oxidative Damage Assay**)

- MAOA or COMT SNPs (**DNA Methylation Pathway**)

References:

American Association for Clinical Chemistry (2010)
Urine Metanephrines
http://labtestsonline.org/understanding/analytes/urine-metanephrine/tab/sample/
Accessed 04 Aug 2014

Daubner, S Colette; Le, Tiffany; Wang, Shanzhi (2011)
Tyrosine hydroxylase and regulation of dopamine synthesis.
Archives of biochemistry and biophysics vol. 508 (1) p. 1-12

Eisenhofer, Graeme; Kopin, Irwin J.; Goldstein, David S. (2004)
Catecholamine Metabolism: A Contemporary View with Implications for Physiology and Medicine
Pharmacol. Rev. vol. 56 (3) p. 331-349

Eisenhofer, Graeme (2001)
Free or Total Metanephrines for Diagnosis of Pheochromocytoma: What Is the Difference?
Clin. Chem. vol. 47 (6) p. 988-989

Goldstein, David S (2010)
Catecholamines 101.
Clinical autonomic research: official journal of the Clinical Autonomic Research Society vol. 20 (6) p. 331-52

Goldstein, David S.; Eisenhofer, Graeme; Kopin, Irwin J. (2003)
Sources and Significance of Plasma Levels of Catechols and Their Metabolites in Humans
J. Pharmacol. Exp. Ther. vol. 305 (3) p. 800-811

Jong, Wilhelmina H. A. de; Eisenhofer, Graeme; Post, Wendy J.; Muskiet, Frits A. J.; Vries, Elisabeth G. E. de et al. (2013)
Dietary Influences on Plasma and Urinary Metanephrines: Implications for Diagnosis of Catecholamine-Producing Tumors
Endocrine Society

Merke, Deborah P. MD, et al. (2000)
Adrenomedullary Dysplasia and Hypofunction in Patients with Classic 21-Hydroxylase Deficiency
N Engl J Med 2000; 343:1362-1368
November 9, 2000

Oeltmann, Timothy; Carson, Robert; Shannon, John R.; Ketch, Terry; Robertson, David (2004)
Assessment of O-methylated catecholamine levels in plasma and urine for diagnosis of autonomic disorders
Autonomic Neuroscience vol. 116 (1) p. 1-10

Wong, Dona L; Tai, T C; Wong-Faull, David C; Claycomb, Robert; Kvetnanský, Richard (2008)
Adrenergic responses to stress: transcriptional and post-transcriptional changes.
Annals of the New York Academy of Sciences vol. 1148 p. 249-56

Adrenal and paraganglia tumors

Rare catecholamine-secreting tumors may occur in the adrenal medulla (pheochromocytoma) and elsewhere in the body (extra-adrenal paraganglioma). About 90% of pheochromocytomae are located in the adrenal glands. While a few are cancerous, most are benign – they do not spread beyond their original location – although most do continue to grow. Paragangliomae have been found in the abdomen, chest, neck and head; they may develop anywhere there are sympathetic nerve cells. Depending on the location and type of tumor, excess epinephrine, norepinephrine or occasionally, dopamine, may be secreted. Metanephrine, normetanephrine and 3-methoxytyramine measurements are considered superior to epinephrine and norepinephrine for the evaluation of these tumors, because most catecholamines are metabolized in the cells that produce them. Catecholamines produced in the tumor undergo metabolism continuously by the enzyme catechol-O-methyltransferase (COMT), even if they do not reach the bloodstream.

Most pheochromocytomae secrete predominantly norepinephrine. Paragangliomae may secrete norepinephrine in an intermittent, uncontrolled manner, which may cause serious health problems including stroke, heart attack, and even death. The differences in catecholamine secretion reflects differences in the expression of catecholamine biosynthetic and metabolic enzymes and can explain differences in presenting symptoms. Paroxysmal hypertension and symptoms such as palpitations, anxiety, dyspnea (shortness of breath), and hyperglycemia may be more common in patients with pheochromocytomae producing primarily epinephrine. Symptoms usually occur in discrete, intermittent attacks and usually last 15 to 20 minutes. The attacks may increase in frequency, length, and severity as the tumor grows. Left untreated, the symptoms may worsen as the tumor grows and, over a period of time, the hypertension may cause kidney damage, heart disease, and raise the risk of a stroke or heart attack. Other symptoms may occur less frequently and include:

- Abdominal pain
- Chest pain
- Irritability
- Nervousness
- Pallor
- Sweating
- Weight loss
- Hand tremor
- Insomnia

Inheritance of the following conditions may predispose patients for catecholamine-secreting tumors:

- Multiple endocrine neoplasia
- *http://ghr.nlm.nih.gov/condition/ multiple-endocrine-neoplasia*
- Sturge-Weber *http://www.ninds.nih. gov/disorders/sturge_weber/sturge_ weber.htm*
- von Hippel Lindau
- *http://ghr.nlm.nih.gov/condition/ von-hippel-lindau-syndrome*
- von Recklinghausen (neurofibromatosis) *http:// www.ninds.nih.gov/disorders/ neurofibromatosis/neurofibromatosis. htm*

Solitary increases in methoxytyramine indicate dopamine-secreting tumors. These tumors characterize 70% of patients with succinate dehydrogenase SDHB and SDHD genetic mutations.

Patients with catecholamine-secreting tumors virtually always have high plasma normetanephrine or metanephrine levels, reflecting metabolism of norepinephrine or epinephrine in the tumor before release of the catecholamines into the circulation. Plasma levels of metanephrines (normetanephrine and metanephrine) constitute the most sensitive blood test to detect these tumors.

24-hour urine tests may not always be successful in detecting an intermittently secreting tumor, and are considered confirmational tests for plasma results.

References:

A.D.A.M. Medical Encyclopedia (2012)
PubMed Health
*http://www.ncbi.nlm.nih.gov/pubmedhealth/
PMH0001380/*
Accessed 04 December 2014

American Association for Clinical Chemistry (2013) Urine Metanephrines.
*http://labtestsonline.org/understanding/
analytes/urine-metanephrine/tab/sample/*
Accessed 25 July 2014.

American Association of Endocrine Surgeons (2013)
Paraganglioma (adrenaline-producing tumor outside the adrenal gland)
http://endocrinediseases.org/adrenal/paraganglioma.shtml
Accessed 04 December 2014

Eisenhofer, Graeme; Lenders, Jacques W.M.; Timmers, Henri; Mannelli, Massimo; Grebe, Stefan K. et al. (2011)
Measurements of Plasma Methoxytyramine, Normetanephrine, and Metanephrine as Discriminators of Different Hereditary Forms of Pheochromocytoma
Clin. Chem. vol. 57 (3) p. 411-420

Foo, S.H.; Chan, S.P.; Ananda, V.; Rajasingam V. (2010)
Dopamine-secreting phaeochromo-cytomas and paragangliomas: clinical features and management
Singapore Med J 2010; 51(5) : e89

Gupta, Pallav, MD. (2004)
Adrenal gland and paraganglia
*http://www.pathologyoutlines.com/topic/
adrenalpheochromocytoma.html*
Accessed 04 December 2014

Goldstein, David S.; Eisenhofer, Graeme; Kopin, Irwin J. (2003)
Sources and Significance of Plasma Levels of Catechols and Their Metabolites in Humans
J. Pharmacol. Exp. Ther. vol. 305 (3) p. 800-811

Serotonin (5-hydroxytryptamine)

Serotonin signaling in the central nervous system (CNS) may influence mood, appetite, sleep, memory and learning, homeostasis, and sexual behaviors. Serotonin may modulate the activity or release of other neurotransmitters. Approximately 10% of plasma serotonin is synthesized in the central nervous system.

There are a great many serotonin receptors with different levels of affinity, expression and function that may also play a role in disorders of serotonin metabolism. Serotonin affects vasoconstriction and vasodilation. Serotonin is also essential for gastrointestinal health; 95% of the body's serotonin is found in the gut. Osteoblasts (bone cells) have serotonin receptors and studies indicates that serotonin levels may affect bone mass. Animal studies indicate that serotonin signaling may promote liver regeneration. Research continues to discover how serotonin signaling further regulates physiological functions.

Effects:

Decreased serotonin levels have been associated with obsessive-compulsive disorder (OCD), anger, insomnia, and depression. Some eating disorders and migraine headaches may also be related to low serotonin levels. Low levels of serotonin have been associated with aggressive behavior in animal studies. One study of pregnant women has associated low urinary serotonin levels with increased risk of premature birth. Low levels of both serotonin and low 5-hydrosyindoleacetic acid (5-HIAA) in cerebrospinal fluid have been associated in studies with a type of depression more likely to suicide. There is currently no simple, direct correlation of serotonin or norepinephrine levels in the brain and mood. Studies indicate, however, that serotonin depletion is more likely to affect mood in those with a family history of mood disorders. There may be a gender-related difference in response to serotonin; PET scans demonstrate that, compared to men, women had significantly higher 5-HT1A serotonin receptor and lower 5-HTT serotonin transporter binding potentials in most brain regions. Women also produce less serotonin than men. Mutations or single nucleotide polymorphisms (SNPs), in enzymes may affect serotonin synthesis, metabolism or receptor function. Several SNPs have been identified and linked to depression; research continues in this area.

Both enterocytes and osteoblasts possess serotonin receptors. In the peripheral nervous system, low levels of serotonin may affect gastrointestinal (GI) motility, and possibly bone mass. Low serotonin levels have been associated with irritable bowel syndrome. Inhibition of serotonin synthesis has been shown experimentally to increase bone mass. Serotonin is also converted into melatonin; low levels of melatonin may affect circadian rhythms, sleep patterns and GI motility. Medications that may decrease serotonin and 5-HIAA levels include aspirin, ethyl alcohol, imipramine, levodopa, monoamine oxidase inhibitors (MAOIs), heparin, isoniazid, methyldopa, and tricyclic anti-

depressants. Low serotonin levels may induce cravings for carbohydrates.

Excess serotonin may contribute to symptoms of schizophrenia. Current research indicates that excess neurotransmitter or receptor function in both dopamine and serotonin pathways may contribute to schizophrenia. Serotonin levels may be increased by exercise, increased daylight (or daylight equivalent) exposure, low-protein high-carbohydrate meals, insulin or by tryptophan or 5-hydroxytryptophan (5-HTP) supplements. Some studies indicate that therapeutic massage may also elevate serotonin levels. Plasma and CNS levels of tryptophan are increased during carbohydrate-rich, protein-poor meals or due to increased plasma insulin levels. A study demonstrated elevated plasma levels of serotonin, its metabolite 5-hydroxyindoleacetic acid (5-HIAA), and urine albumin in and Asian population of men with Type II diabetes. Exogenous estrogens have been shown to elevate both serotonin and 5-HIAA levels in post-menopausal women.

Serotonin is converted into melatonin by the enzyme arylalkylamine N-acetyltransferase; deficient function of this enzyme may result in elevated serotonin and low melatonin levels. Deficient function of the serotonin transporter (SERT) may prevent normal reuptake of serotonin by pre-synaptic neurons, and result in elevated serotonin levels. Single nucleotide polymorphisms (SNPs) may affect SERT function.

Serotonin Syndrome is an excess of serotonin due to a sudden change in serotonin re-uptake function. The change in serotonin reuptake is usually due to a new medication, such as a serotonin re-uptake inhibitor (SSRI) or a monoamine oxidase inhibitor (MAOI). Symptoms of serotonin excess are wide-ranging. A triad of symptoms including altered mental status, neuromuscular hyperactivity or hyperreflexia, and autonomic instability, is suspicious for serotonin excess. Symptoms of Serotonin Syndrome include:

- Confusion

- Agitation

- Restlessness

- Dilated pupils

- Headache

- Changes in blood pressure, temperature

- Nausea or vomiting

- Diarrhea

- Rapid heart rate

- Tremor

- Loss of muscle coordination

- Twitching muscles

- Shivering and goose bumps

- Heavy sweating

The main diseases that may be associated with measurable increases in serotonin are neuroectodermal tumors, in particular, carcinoid tumors arising from GI enterochromaffin cells. The enzyme 5-HTP decarboxylase, which converts the intermediate 5-HTP to serotonin, is present in midgut tumors. About 70% of cases are midgut carcinoids (tumors are found within the jejunum, ileum, or appendix). Only about 10% of midgut carcinoids produce enough serotonin to cause symptoms. Diagnosis of carcinoid tumor requires evaluation of multiple biomarkers:

- plasma serotonin

- urine serotonin

- urine 5-HIAA (HIAA / 5-Hydroxyindoleacetic Acid)

- serum chromogranin A

Urine serotonin is the least likely marker to be elevated, and is not, in isolation, considered diagnostic for carcinoid tumors. Urine and plasma levels of serotonin and 5-HIAA may vary with the inclusion of foods rich in serotonin or the use of medications that increase serotonin levels. Foods including avocados, bananas, pineapples, plums, walnuts, tomatoes, kiwi fruit, and eggplant may interfere with serotonin and 5-HIAA testing and should be avoided for 3 days prior to and during urine collection. Medications that may increase 5-HIAA include acetaminophen, caffeine, ephedrine, diazepam (Valium), nicotine, glyceryl guaiacolate (guaifenisin), and phenobarbital. 5-HT receptor antagonists may also elevate serotonin and 5-HIAA levels.

Serotonin and Migraine

Research continues into the origin of migraine headaches. Evidence indicates that dysregulation of serotonin synthesis and signaling in certain areas of the brain may contribute to the causation of migraine headaches. The current understanding of the relationship between serotonin and migraine headaches includes:

- Migraineurs are predominantly female

  - There are gender differences in serotonin transporters in the midbrain and in peripheral platelet cells

- Men synthesize serotonin faster, and with left/right brain differences compared to females
- Serotonin reactivity, when experimentally induced in hand veins, is greater in women than men
- Though reserves are similar in men and women, women seem to use up reserves more quickly when stressed
- Acute tryptophan depletion results in a larger decrease in serotonin synthesis in women
- Migraine triggers may include hormonal changes (peri-menstrual), post-stress ("weekend" headache), alcohol, pain and after intense emotion/alarm/fear

- Seasonal variation is seen in migraine frequency; a study in an Artic population reported peak migraine frequency in January, and lowest migraine frequency in June

  - Early evidence indicates that the vitamin D response element (VDRE), in combination with vitamin D, increases the expression of the synthesis enzyme tryptophan hydroxylase in the brain

Synthesis and Metabolism:

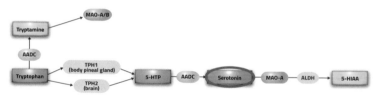

Serotonin is synthesized from the amino acid L-tryptophan in pre-synaptic neurons. The enzyme tryptophan hydroxylase (TPH) produces 5-hydroxytryptophan (5-HTP) which is converted to serotonin by aromatic amino acid decarboxylase (AADC), also called 5-HTP decarboxylase. AADC is pyridoxal-phosphate (B6) dependent. Different forms of the TPH enzyme are found in the brain and in the gastrointestinal system. Evidence indicates that vitamin D upregulates the expression of TPH2 in the brain and inhibits the expression of TPH1 in the periphery.

A specific sequence of DNA of the vitamin D response element (VDRE), which is located near vitamin D-regulated genes, is involved in vitamin D signaling. Once synthesized, serotonin is either stored in neuron vesicles or metabolized by monoamine oxidase A (MAO-A). Serotonin is unable to cross the blood-brain barrier (BBB) and must be synthesized both peripherally and in the central nervous system. Most peripheral production occurs in the gastrointestinal (GI) enterochromaffin cells. The gastrointestinal tract produces about 80% of the body's serotonin. Serotonin released into the synapse is taken back up into presynaptic neurons by the serotonin transporter (SERT). There may be multiple forms of SERT (isoforms) in the body and nervous system. Platelets take up 10% of plasma Serotonin. High levels of serotonin within the platelet cells is a consistent finding in autistic patients. Low levels of platelet serotonin have been associated with depression and anemia. The serotonin released when platelets aggregate may contribute to vasoconstriction and the symptoms of metabolic syndrome in some populations.

Under physiological conditions only about 5% of L-tryptophan is metabolized to serotonin. The complex interaction of the GI microbiome, the immune system and the cells of the intestine all have an influence on serotonin synthesis, release, and degradation. A recent study indicated that the probiotc *Bifidobacteria infantis* may modulate tryptophan metabolism. The proportions of dietary tryptophan and phenylalanine that enter the circulation are limited by three hepatic enzymes that destroy them on the hepatic first pass to prevent elevated plasma levels. During the "first pass" through hepatic circulation, the liver metabolizes 30-80% of GI serotonin to 5-hydroxyindolacetic acid (5-HIAA). Serotonin may also be converted to 5-HIAA in the lungs.

Tryptophan may also be converted into kynurenine by another enzymatic pathway. The shift of tryptophan metabolism away from serotonin towards kynureneine may be promoted by increased cortisol, inflammation or bacterial lipopolysaccharide ("endotoxin"). Aging and oxidative stress may also upregulate the kynurenine pathway. Accumulation of kynurenic acid, an N-methyl-D-aspartate (NMDA) receptor antagonist, has been associated with symptoms of schizophrenia and cognitive degeneration.

Serotonin increases GI blood flow, motility, and fluid secretion. Alterations in tissue levels and the mucosal production of serotonin is common in a variety of gastrointestinal disorders; research is ongoing to determine the effects that these alterations may have on plasma and urine serotonin levels. In the gut, serotonin signaling contributes to the regulation of peristalsis and gut motility. Loss of TPH function (serotonin synthesis) in the serotonin neurons of the gut may result in accelerated gastric emptying, but decreased overall GI transit time and poor intestinal peristalsis. Loss of GI serotonin neuron signaling is thought to contribute to irritable bowel syndrome. Increased GI serotonin has been associated with nausea, vomiting, Celiac disease, inflammatory bowel disease (IBD) and irritable bowel syndrome with diarrhea (IBS-D). An elevation in serotonin after meals has been associated with dyspepsia and IBS-D. In some studies, irritable bowel syndrome with constipation (IBS-C) and prolonged transit time has been associated with impaired serotonin response after meals; for some patients there may be a response to 5-HT4 agonist medications.

Thyroid function may affect serotonin signaling. Human and animal studies indicate that increasing levels of thyroid hormone may increase CNS serotonin levels, serotonin signaling and may desensitize 5-HT_{1A} and sensitize 5-HT_2 receptors. Animal studies indicate that hypothyroid conditions may decrease levels of serotonin, its precursor 5-hydroxytryptophan (5-HTP) and it's metabolite 5-hydroxyindoleacetic acid (5-HIAA). These thyroid-induced changes seem to be specific to certain areas of the brain. Animal studies indicate that exogenous (supplemental) thyroid hormone (T3) increase 5-HTP, serotonin and 5-HIAA; such effects may require chronic administration of thyroid hormone. Human studies indicate that MAO activity may decrease in hyperthyroid conditions, and normalize with with normal thyroid hormone levels.

Urine and plasma levels of serotonin may vary with the intake of certain foods rich in serotonin and medications that either increase or decrease serotonin levels.

Receptors:

Serotonin receptors (5HT-receptors) have a variety of functions. There are multiple 5-HT receptor sub-types in each of the seven 5-HT receptor families. Most 5-HT activity is the result of second messenger signaling through cyclic adenosine monophosphate (cAMP) or phosphorylation of proteins. At least two serotonin receptors $5HT_{1B}$ and $5HT_{1D}$ act as auto-receptors to regulate the synthesis and release of serotonin from neurons. $5\text{-}HT_{1A}$ and $5\text{-}HT_{1B}$ are found in pre-synaptic neurons and may modulate serotonin release. Mutations or single nucleotide polymorphisms (SNPs) may affect receptor conformation or function. 5-HT receptor information has been compiled from animal, in vitro and genetics studies.

$5\text{-}HT_1$ receptors

- decrease neuron excitability (action potential or likelihood of firing)
- $5\text{-}HT_{1A}$ may be associated with neuropsychiatric disorders such as anxiety, depression or schizophrenia
- $5\text{-}HT_{1B}$ may regulate the release of other neurotransmitters; may affect motor function, behavior, cognition

$5\text{-}HT_2$ receptors

- increase neuron excitability
- $5\text{-}HT_2$ may be associated with depression, cognition, sleep, schizophrenia, reward behavior/addiction

- $5\text{-}HT_2$ A has been associated with anxiety disorders and migraine with aura
- mediates vasoconstriction

$5\text{-}HT_3$ receptors

- ionotropic channels for sodium, potassium and calcium (the balance of ions inside and outside of a neuron determines its action potential)
- alters GI motility and vomiting; modulates release of GABA and serototonin
- function may be modified by anesthetics, alcohol or neuroactive steroids
- gonadal steroids (sex hormones) have been shown in vitro to antagonize $5\text{-}HT_3$ receptors

$5\text{-}HT_4$ receptors

- increase neuron excitability
- modulates GI motility
- may modulate cardiac function
- may be associated with learning, memory and anxiety

$5\text{-}HT_5$ receptors

- decrease neuron excitability; research continues into $5\text{-}HT_5$ function

$5\text{-}HT_6$ receptors

- increase neuron excitability;
- studies indicate that $5\text{-}HT_6$ may regulate glutamatergic and cholinergic neuronal activity
- may be associated with depression, anxiety, schizophrenia, cognition, epilepsy

- may be associated with stress response

$5\text{-}HT_7$ receptors

- increase neuron excitability

- studies indicate $5\text{-}HT_7$ mediates the relaxation of smooth muscle in GI tract and cardiovascular system

- may regulate circadian rhythms and sleep

- may be associated with depression, schizophrenia, cognition, sleep, epilepsy

The serotonin signaling system may be affected by antihypertensive, antidepressant, anti-anxiety and anti-psychotic medications. These medications act upon one or more of the 5-HT receptors.

Consider:

- Essential precursor Tryptophan status (**Plasma** or **Urine Amino Acids**)

- Gastrointestinal function (**Comprehensive Stool Analysis**)

- Glutathione status (**Glutathione; erythrocytes**)

- Bacterial lipopolysaccharide (LPS) (**Intestinal Permeability Test**)

- Oxidative stress (**DNA Oxidative Damage Assay/8-OHdG**)

- MAOA or COMT SNPs (**DNA Methylation Pathway**)

References:

Barnes, Nicholas M. and Neumaier, John F. (2011)
Neuronal 5-HT Receptors and SERT
University of Birmingham Medical School

Bauer, M.; Heinz, A.; Whybrow, P.C.(2002)
Thyroid hormones, serotonin and mood: of synergy and significance in the adult brain
Nature Publishing Group vol. 7 (2)

Cansev, M.; Wurtman, R.J. (2007) Chapter 4 Aromatic Amino Acids in the Brain
Handbook of Neurochemistry and Molecular Neurobiology
Springer, US.

De Maeyer, J H; Lefebvre, R A; Schuurkes, J A J (2008)
5-HT4 receptor agonists: similar but not the same.
Neurogastroenterology and motility : the official journal of the European Gastrointestinal Motility Society vol. 20 (2) p. 99-112

Field, Tiffany; Hernandez-Reif, Maria; Diego, Miguel; Schanberg, Saul; Kuhn, Cynthia (2009)
CORTISOL DECREASES AND SEROTONIN AND DOPAMINE INCREASE FOLLOWING MASSAGE THERAPY
Informa UK Ltd UK

Field, Tiffany; Diego, Miguel; Hernandez-Reif, Maria; Figueiredo, Barbara; Deeds, Osvelia et al. (2008)
Prenatal serotonin and neonatal outcome: brief report.
Infant behavior & development vol. 31 (2) p. 316-20

Fink, Klaus B. and Göthert, Manfred. (2007)
5-HT Receptor Regulation of Neurotransmitter Release
Pharmacological Reviews December 2007 vol. 59 no. 4 360-417

Fukui, Michiaki; Tanaka, Muhei; Toda, Hitoshi; Asano, Mai; Yamazaki, Masahiro et al. (2012)
High plasma 5-hydroxyindole-3-acetic acid concentrations in subjects with metabolic syndrome.
Diabetes care vol. 35 (1) p. 163-7

Gershon, Michael D (2013)

5-Hydroxytryptamine (serotonin) in the gastrointestinal tract.
Current opinion in endocrinology, diabetes, and obesity vol. 20 (1) p. 14-21

Hannon, Jason; Hoyer, Daniel (2008)
Molecular biology of 5-HT receptors.
Behavioural brain research vol. 195 (1) p. 198-213

Iqbal, Mohammad M. MD, MPH, MSPH
Overview of serotonin syndrome.
ANNALS OF CLINICAL PSYCHIATRY 2012;24(4):310-318

Janusonis, Skirmantas (2005)
Statistical distribution of blood serotonin as a predictor of early autistic brain abnormalities.
Theoretical biology & medical modelling vol. 2 p. 27

Jovanovic, Hristina; Lundberg, Johan; Karlsson, Per; Cerin, Åsta; Saijo, Tomoyuki et al. (2008)
Sex differences in the serotonin 1A receptor and serotonin transporter binding in the human brain measured by PET
NeuroImage vol. 39 (3) p. 1408-1419

Lippert, Theodor H.; Filshie, Marcus; Mück, Alfred O.; Seeger, Harald; Zwirner, Manfred (1996)
Serotonin metabolite excretion after post-menopausal estradiol therapy
Maturitas vol. 24 (1) p. 37-41

Oxenkrug, Gregory F (2010)
Tryptophan kynurenine metabolism as a common mediator of genetic and environmental impacts in major depressive disorder: the serotonin hypothesis revisited
40 years later.
The Israel journal of psychiatry and related sciences vol. 47 (1) p. 56-63

Panconesi, Alessandro (2008)
Serotonin and migraine: a reconsideration of the central theory.
The journal of headache and pain vol. 9 (5) p. 267-76

Ruljancic, Nedjeljka; Mihanovic, Mate; Cepelak, Ivana; Bakliza, Ana; Curkovic, Katarina Dodig (2013)
Platelet serotonin and magnesium concentrations in suicidal and non-suicidal depressed patients.
Magnesium research : official organ of the International Society for the Development of Research on Magnesium vol. 26 (1) p. 9-17

Spiller, R (2007)
Recent advances in understanding the role of serotonin in gastrointestinal motility in functional bowel disorders: alterations in 5-HT signalling and metabolism in human disease.
Neurogastroenterology and motility : the official journal of the European Gastrointestinal Motility Society vol. 19 Suppl 2 p. 25-31

Srinivasan, Venkatramanujam; Spence, D Warren; Pandi-Perumal, Seithikurippu R; Brown, Gregory M; Cardinali, Daniel P (2011)
Melatonin in mitochondrial dysfunction and related disorders.
International journal of Alzheimer's disease vol. 2011 p. 326320

Thomas, David R; Hagan, Jim J (2004)
5-HT7 receptors.
Current drug targets. CNS and neurological disorders vol. 3 (1) p. 81-90

Woolley, Marie L; Marsden, Charles A; Fone, Kevin C F (2004)
5-ht6 receptors.
Current drug targets. CNS and neurological disorders vol. 3 (1) p. 59-79

Wang, Mingde (2011)
Neurosteroids and GABA-A Receptor Function.
Frontiers in endocrinology vol. 2 p. 44

Young, Simon N (2007)
How to increase serotonin in the human brain without drugs.
Journal of psychiatry & neuroscience : JPN vol. 32 (6) p. 394-9

5-hydroxyindoleacetic acid (5-HIAA)

5-hydroxyindoleacetic acid (5-HIAA) is a metabolite of serotonin. Clinically, urinary 5-HIAA is an indicator of serotonin synthesis and metabolism. Levels of serotonin and 5-HIAA may be affected by a variety of factors. Ninety-five percent of the body's serotonin is found in the gut.

Effects:

Decreased levels (2 mg/24 hr) of urinary 5-HIAA have been associated with depression, Hartnup disease, mastocytosis, phenylketonuria, renal disease or small bowel resection. Low levels of tryptophan or serotonin may result in low levels of 5-HIAA. Medications that may decrease 5-HIAA include aspirin, ethyl alcohol, imipramine, levodopa, MAO inhibitors, heparin, isoniazid, methyldopa, and tricyclic antidepressants.

Excess 5-HIAA has been associated with Celiac disease and chronic renal insufficiency. A study demonstrated elevated plasma levels of serotonin, its metabolite 5-hydroxyindolacetic acid (5-HIAA), and urine albumin in and Asian population of men with Type II diabetes. Exogenous estrogens have been shown to elevate both serotonin and 5-HIAA levels in post-menopausal women. Serotonin is converted into melatonin by the enzyme arylalkylamine N-acetyltransferase; deficient function of this enzyme may result in elevated serotonin and 5-HIAA levels and low melatonin levels. Deficient function of the serotonin transporter (SERT) may prevent normal reuptake of serotonin by pre-synaptic neurons, and result in elevated serotonin and 5-HIAA levels.

Serotonin Syndrome is an excess of serotonin due to a sudden change in serotonin re-uptake function. The change in serotonin reuptake is usually due to a new medication, such as a serotonin re-uptake inhibitor (SSRI) or a monoamine oxidase inhibitor (MAOI). Symptoms of serotonin excess are wide-ranging. A triad of symptoms including altered mental status, neuromuscular hyperactivity or hyper-reflexia, and autonomic instability, is suspicious for serotonin excess. Symptoms of Serotonin Syndrome include:

- Confusion
- Agitation
- Restlessness
- Dilated pupils
- Headache
- Changes in blood pressure, temperature
- Nausea or vomiting
- Diarrhea
- Rapid heart rate
- Tremor
- Loss of muscle coordination
- Twitching muscles
- Shivering and goose bumps
- Heavy sweating

The main disease that may be associated with measurable increases in 5-HIAA is carcinoid tumors arising from GI enterochromaffin cells. The enzyme 5-HTP decarboxylase, which converts the intermediate 5-hydroxytryptophan (5-HTP) to serotonin, is present in midgut tumors. About 70% of cases are midgut carcinoids (tumors are found within the jejunum, ileum, or appendix). Only about 10% of midgut carcinoids produce enough serotonin to cause symptoms. Levels of over 25 mg/24 hr (131 umol/day) may indicate large carcinoid tumors of the duodenum, ileum, biliary tree or pancreas.

Levels of 7-25 mg/24 hr have been associated with Celiac disease, tropical sprue, Cystic fibrosis, foregut carcinoid tumors, midgut carcinoid tumors, carcinoma of the bronchus, Whipple disease and ovarian carcinoid tumours. Foregut carcinoid tumors may arise from the respiratory tract, stomach, pancreas, or duodenum. Midgut carcinoid tumors may arise from the within jejunum, ileum, or appendix. Diagnosis of carcinoid tumor requires the evaluation of multiple biomarkers:

- serotonin

- urine serotonin

- urine 5-HIAA

- serum chromogranin A

Urine and plasma levels of 5-HIAA may vary with the inclusion of foods rich in serotonin or the use of medications that increase serotonin levels.

Foods, including avocados, bananas, pineapples, plums, walnuts, tomatoes, kiwi fruit, and eggplant may interfere with 5-HIAA testing and should be avoided for 3 days prior to and during urine collection. Medications that may increase 5-HIAA include acetaminophen, caffeine, ephedrine, diazepam (Valium), nicotine, glyceryl guaiacolate (guaifenisin), and phenobarbital. 5-HT receptor antagonists may also elevate 5-HIAA levels.

Synthesis and Metabolism:

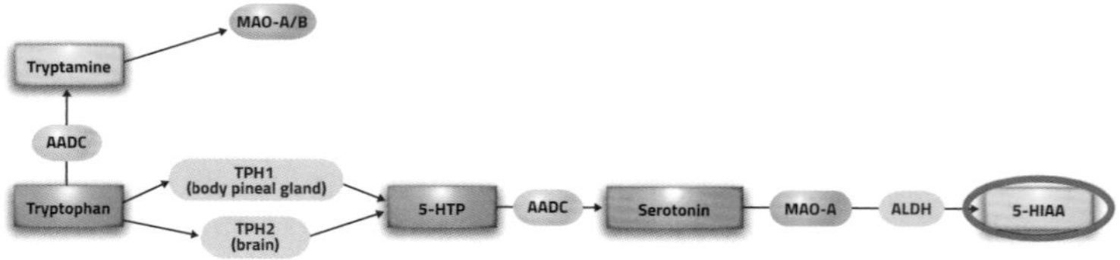

Serotonin is synthesized from the amino acid L-tryptophan in presynaptic neurons. The enzyme tryptophan hydroxylase (TPH) produces 5-hydroxytryptophan (5-HTP) which is converted to serotonin by 5-HTP decarboxylase. Once synthesized, serotonin is either stored in neuron vesicles or metabolized by monoamine oxidase A (MAO-A) into 5-HIAA. 5-HIAA levels represent about 1% of the tryptophan metabolized in the body. Low levels of tryptophan may result in low levels of serotonin and 5-HIAA. Most peripheral serotonin

production occurs in the gastrointestinal (GI) enterochromaffin cells. The gastrointestinal tract produces about 80% of the body's serotonin. The complex interaction of the microbiome, the immune system and the mucosa of the intestine all have an influence on serotonin synthesis, release, and degradation.

Serotonin released into the synapse is taken back up into presynaptic neurons by the serotonin transporter (SERT). There may be multiple forms of SERT (isoforms) in the body and nervous system. Deficient function of the serotonin transporter (SERT) may prevent normal reuptake of serotonin by pre-synaptic neurons, and result in elevated serotonin and 5-HIAA levels. Platelets take up 10% of plasma serotonin. The serotonin released when platelets aggregate may contribute to vasoconstriction and the symptoms of metabolic syndrome in some populations. During the "first pass" through hepatic circulation, the liver metabolizes 30-80% of GI serotonin to 5-hydroxyindoleacetic acid (5-HIAA). Serotonin may also be converted to 5-HIAA in the lungs. Serotonin is converted into melatonin by the enzyme arylalkylamine N-acetyltransferase; deficient function of this enzyme may result in elevated serotonin and 5-HIAA levels and low melatonin levels.

Receptors:

5-HIAA is not known to bind with neurotransmitter receptors.

Consider:

- MAO-A SNPs (DNA Methylation Pathway)

References:

American Association for Clinical Chemistry
www.labtestsonline.org
Accessed 19 December 2014

Fukui, Michiaki; Tanaka, Muhei; Toda, Hitoshi; Asano, Mai; Yamazaki, Masahiro et al. (2012)
High plasma 5-hydroxyindole-3-acetic acid concentrations in subjects with metabolic syndrome.
Diabetes care vol. 35 (1) p. 163-7

Fukui, Michiaki; Ose, Hiroyuki; Hasegawa, Goji; Yoshikawa, Toshikazu; Nakamura, Naoto (2007)
Association Between Urinary Albumin Excretion and Plasma 5-Hydroxyindole-

3-Acetic Acid Concentration in Men With Type 2 Diabetes
Diabetes Care vol. 30 (10) p. 2649-2651

Garg, Shivani, MBBS, MD and Staros, Eric B, MD
5-hydroxyindole acetic acid (5-HIAA)
http://emedicine.medscape.com/article/2089202-overview retrieved 02 Sept 2014

Manocha, Marcus; Khan, Waliul I (2012)
Serotonin and GI Disorders: An Update on Clinical and Experimental Studies
American College of Gastroenterology vol. 3 p. e13

Sebekova K, Spustova V, Opatrny K Jr., Dzurik R (2001)
Serotonin and 5-hydroxyindole-acetic acid
Bratisl Lek Listy 2001; 102 (8): 351.356

Spiller, R (2007)
Recent advances in understanding the role of serotonin in gastrointestinal motility in functional bowel disorders: alterations in 5-HT signalling and metabolism in human disease.
Neurogastroenterology and motility : the official journal of the European Gastrointestinal Motility Society vol. 19 Suppl 2 p. 25-31

Tryptamine

Tryptamine is derived from the essential amino acid tryptophan. Tryptamine and other "trace amines" are found at very low (nanmolar) levels in nerve cells. The interaction of trace amines, and their receptors, in the brain may play a role in psychiatric and neurological disease processes. Experimental evidence suggests that dysregulation of trace amines may alter levels of dopamine, norepinephrine or serotonin, and thereby contribute to neuropsychiatric disorders such as attention deficit hyperactivity disorder (ADHD), schizophrenia, depression and neurodegenerative diseases. Tryptamine levels may affect artery resistance (vasoconstriction) and serotonin signaling. Inhibitory effects of serotonin may be potentiated by tryptamine. Clinically, trace amines are generally considered sympathomimetic (they mimic the action of sympathetic nerve stimulation), they may affect vasoconstriction and blood pressure. In large, supra-physiologic doses, the effects of trace amines are similar to amphetamines.

Effects:

Decreased tryptamine levels or deficient trace amine functions may be associated with some depressive disorders. Aromatic amino acid decarboxylase (AADC) metabolizes tyrosine, tryptophan into the trace amines tyramine and tryptamine. Activation of monoamine neurotransmitter receptors (via receptor agonists or electrical stimulation) decreases AADC activity and trace amine levels. Reserpine may deplete CNS levels of trace amines. Multiple studies demonstrate that loss of neurons in specific brain areas or loss of specific types of neurons may result in decreased trace amine levels. Loss of D-neurons containing AADC has been associated with some forms of schizophrenia. The function of both trace amine–associated receptors (TAARs) and the level of trace amines are thought to contribute

to altered brain activity. Low levels of tryptamine may result if the level of the precursor amino acid tryptophan is deficient.

Excess tryptamine and increased AADC activity have been associated with some forms of schizophrenia. Increases in AADC activity may increase trace amine levels, without affecting levels of monoamine neurotransmitters. Decreased monoamine neurotransmitter receptor activation (receptor antagonists, neurotransmitter depletion) may result in an increase in AADC activity and increased trace amine levels. Urinary tryptamine levels seem to correlate with symptom severity in schizophrenia. Methylated tryptamines may also play a role in the development of schizophrenia. Methylated tryptamines, such as N,N-dimethyltryptamine (DMT), are produced within the body, and may have hallucinogenic effects.

Trace amines may be generated in the gastrointestinal tract by protein-fermenting gut bacteria after a protein-rich meal, and they may be found in a variety of foods as the result of food spoilage or deliberate fermentation. Dietary trace amines are usually metabolized quickly by MAO enzymes. Elevated levels of trace amines may occur due to phenylketonuria, ergot poisoning or the use of MAO inhibitors.

Synthesis and Metabolism:

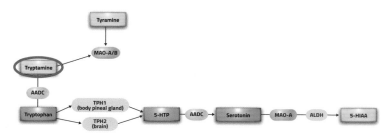

The function of aromatic L-amino acid decarboxylase (AADC) is the rate-limiting step for tryptamine synthesis. AADC requires pyridoxal phosphate (vitamin B6) as a cofactor. Altered AADC activity may affect trace amine levels without affecting the levels of monoamine neurotransmitters. Altered AADC activity may, through altered trace amine levels, affect dopamine signaling. Activity is dependent on dopamine levels, but not specific to dopamine. Increased dopamine levels increase AADC activity, which may then affect other neurotransmitter levels.

There is no evidence that tryptamine is stored in vesicles. Trace amines may pass across cell membranes by simple diffusion, and their release may be mediated differently at synapses. Research continues to identify active trace amine transport mechanisms in neurons. Tryptamine is metabolized by monoamine oxidase A and B (MAO) in astroglia and neurons. Animal studies indicate that the addition of selenium and tocopherols to the diet may increase antioxidant capacity and decrease MAO-B activity. Trace amines and their metabolites are excreted by the kidney in urine.

Receptors:

The trace amine-associated receptors (TAARs) are a recently discovered class of receptors that respond to various trace amines. Most TAARs activity is the result of second messenger signaling through cyclic adenosine monophosphate (cAMP) and protein phosphorylation. TAARs are found in the CNS and in the periphery are found in the gastrointestinal tract, lung, and kidneys. In other mammals, some TAARs may serve as olfactory chemoreceptors and may respond to stimulation by odorous amines. Research continues into the function of TAARs and their ligands as not all TAAR subtypes respond to known trace amines. Mutations or single nucleotide polymorphisms in the nine genes coding for TAARs may increase susceptibility risk to schizophrenia or bipolar disorders. *In vitro* and *in vivo* studies indicate:

- TAAR1
  - Intracellular expression
  - Binds to tyramine and PEA with greatest affinity
  - may modulate catecholamines and serotonin by altering cell membrane transport or receptor function
  - Expressed in the CNS and in leukocytes, gastrointestinal tract, lung, and kidneys
    - has been shown in vitro to assist leukocyte chemotaxis towards trace amines; binding of trace amines to TAAR1 in leukocytes has been shown in vitro to promote cytokine release
  - Binds with amphetamines and psychotropic agents (ergot alkaloids, bromocriptine, lisuride, D-lysergic acid diethylamide (LSD), 3,4-methylenedioxymethamphetamine [MDMA or ecstasy])
  - Interacts with the thyroid hormone derivative 3-iodothyronamines, which may affect temperature regulation and cardiac contractility (in vivo)

- TAAR2
  - Has been shown in vitro to assist leukocyte chemotaxis towards trace amines; binding of trace amines to TAAR2 in leukocytes has been shown in vitro to promote cytokine release

- Nonsense mutation may contribute to some cases of schizophrenia

- TAAR5

  - Function and ligand unknown in humans

- TAAR6

  - Expressed in the amygdala of the brain and in leukocytes, kidneys
  - SNP has been associated with increased familial susceptibility to schizophrenia with European or African-American ancestry

  TAAR8

  - Expressed in the amygdala of the brain and in leukocytes, kidneys

- TAAR9

  - Expressed in pituitary and in leukocytes, kidney and skeletal muscle

Trace amines may activate sigma receptors and modulate cellular potassium and calcium channels (in vitro); altering the level of ions inside neurons may change their action potential and firing rate.

Consider:

- Selenium status (**RBC Elements**)

- Glutathione status (**Glutathione; erythrocytes**)

- Oxidative stress (**DNA Oxidative Damage Assay/8-OHdG**)

References:

Anwar, M A; Ford, W R; Broadley, K J; Herbert, A A (2012)
Vasoconstrictor and vasodilator responses to tryptamine of rat-isolated perfused mesentery: comparison with tyramine and -phenylethylamine.
British journal of pharmacology vol. 165 (7) p. 2191-202

Babusyte, Agne; Kotthoff, Matthias; Fiedler, Julia; Krautwurst, Dietmar (2013)
Biogenic amines activate blood leukocytes via trace amine-associated receptors TAAR1 and TAAR2
J. Leukoc. Biol. vol. 93 (3) p. 387-394

Mark D Berry, Mithila R Shitut (2013)
Membrane permeability of trace amines: Evidence for a regulated, activity-dependent, non-exocytotic, synaptic release.
Synapse (New York, N.Y.)

Berry, M.D. (2007)
The Potential of Trace Amines and Their Receptors for Treating Neurological and Psychiatric Diseases
Reviews on Recent Clinical Trials, 2007, 2, 3-19

Berry, Mark D. (2004)
Mammalian central nervous system trace amines. Pharmacologic amphetamines, physiologic neuromodulators.
Journal of Neurochemistry Volume 90, Issue 2, pages 257–271, July 2004

Ledonne, Ada; Berretta, Nicola; Davoli, Alessandro; Rizzo, Giada Ricciardo; Bernardi, Giorgio et al. (2011)
Electrophysiological effects of trace amines on mesencephalic dopaminergic neurons.
Frontiers in systems neuroscience vol. 5 p. 56

Miller, Gregory M (2011)
The emerging role of trace amine-associated receptor 1 in the functional regulation of monoamine transporters and dopaminergic activity.
Journal of Neurochemistry vol. 116 (2) p. 164-76

Narang, Deepak; Tomlinson, Sara; Holt, Andrew; Darrell D. Mousseau, Glen B. Baker, DSc, FCAHS (2011)
Trace amines and their relevance to psychiatry and neurology: a brief overview.

Bulletin of Clinical Psychopharmacology vol. 21 (1) p. 73-79

Tang, Ya-Li; Wang, Shih-Wei; Lin, Shyh-Mirn (2008)
Both inorganic and organic selenium supplements can decrease brain monoamine oxidase B enzyme activity in adult rats. *The British journal of nutrition* vol. 100 (3) p. 660-5

Yu, Ai-Ming; Granvil, Camille P.; Haining, Robert L.; Krausz, Kristopher W.; Corchero, Javier et al. (2003)
The Relative Contribution of Monoamine Oxidase and Cytochrome P450 Isozymes to the Metabolic Deamination of the Trace Amine Tryptamine. *J. Pharmacol. Exp. Ther.* vol. 304 (2) p. 539-546

Zucchi, R; Chiellini, G; Scanlan, T S; Grandy, D K (2006)
Trace amine-associated receptors and their ligands. *British journal of pharmacology* vol. 149 (8) p. 967-78

Glutamate

Glutamate is a non-essential amino acid that may be synthesized in the body or obtained from the diet. It acts as an excitatory neurotransmitter for metabolic and oncogenic (tumor causing) signaling pathways. In the central nervous system (CNS), glutamate is recognized as the primary excitatory neurotransmitter; the glutamate signaling system is involved in fast synaptic transmission between neurons. Glutamate signaling affects neuron maturation, plasticity and higher cognitive functions (mood, memory, behavior). In the periphery, glutamate receptors are found in the gastrointestinal mucosal cells. Animal studies indicate that free glutamate in the gut lumen activates the vagus nerve and stimulates the brain. Glutamate signaling via taste and gut receptors may affect physiologic functions such as digestion, thermoregulation and energy production. Evidence indicates that glutamate excitatory signaling seems uniquely dependent on coordinated activity between CNS astroglia support cells and neurons.

Effects:

Decreased glutamate signaling contributes to apoptosis (self-destruction) of immature neurons. Decreased glutamate signaling has been associated with depressive disorders and psychosis. Research continues into associations between glutamate signaling and cognitive disorders. Disturbances in glutamine metabolism, glutamate synthesis, or amino acid digestion and absorption may affect glutamate levels. Studies using magnetic resonance spectroscopy indicate that astroglia amino acid metabolism may decrease with chronic stress. Decreased function or blockage of N-methyl-D-aspartate (NMDA) receptors may contribute to psychotic symptoms. Reduced glutamate signaling has been associated with elevations in dopamine that may contribute to symptoms of schizophrenia.

Excess activation of glutamate receptors is associated with either neuron necrosis (death) or apoptosis (self-destruction). Excess activation of ionotropic receptors may contribute to neuron degeneration. Glutamate "spillover" from the synaptic cleft both reduces the input specificity of neural signaling and activates extra-synaptic receptors. Excess glutamate signaling, and its effects, has been termed "excitotoxicity", and is considered a contributing factor in the neurodegeneration seen in Huntington's disease, Alzheimer's disease, amyotrophic lateral sclerosis (ALS) and stroke. Animal studies indicate that acute stressors may cause transient elevations in extracellular glutamate, and may temporarily upregulate glutamate receptor expression. Excess glutamate may be associated with defective function of excitatory amino acid transporters (EAATs), glutamine synthetase, the membrane cystine-glutamate antiporter, oxidative stress, hypoxia, tissue injury and increased permeability of the blood brain barrier (BBB).

Evidence indicates that activation of serotonin 5-HT2A receptors may increase the release of glutamate and that psychotic symptoms may occur due to increased stimulation of amino-3-hydroxy-5-methyl-4-isoxazole propionic acid (AMPA) and kainate glutamate receptors. AMPA and kainite receptors are located at the periphery of synapses, and are not normally stimulated if glutamate metabolism, release and re-uptake occur at normal levels.

Synthesis and metabolism:

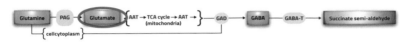

In the CNS astroglia (astrocytes) release of a variety of neuroactive molecules (ATP, D-serine, kynurenic acid), including glutamate, to influence synapse activity. Glial cells are the primary source of glutamate in the CNS; the blood-brain barrier (BBB) prevents the passage of glutamate. Glutamate may be synthesized by astroglia or in the mitochondria of neurons. Glutamate is inter-converted to glutamine through the enzymes glutaminase or glutamine synthetase (both enzymes may have multiple enzyme isoforms). Conversion allows glutamate to be transported into neurons and astroglia as glutamine.

Once synthesized, glutamate is stored in the astroglia and in synaptic vesicles until it is released. Any excess glutamate released into the synapse is cleared by highly efficient excitatory amino acid transporters (EAATs) found on the astroglia. EEATs, unless damaged or defective, keep extracellular glutamate levels low and insufficient for high-affinity glutamate receptor signaling (see Figure 12).

EAAT function is inhibited by reactive oxygen species that are generated within cells as extracellular glutamate levels rise. Extracellular glutamate levels may also increase if glutamine uptake by cells is compromised.

Exposure to excess manganese, a necessary trace element, may disrupt the glutamine/glutamate/GABA cycle. Manganese may compete with iron for transport across the blood brain barrier into the CNS; other transporters may carry manganese across the BBB as well. Excess manganese may disrupt mitochondrial function, increase oxidative stress, and deplete glutathione levels. Manganese tends to concentrate in astroglia mitochondria due to the presence of high-capacity transporters in these cells. Astroglia contribute glutathione, and other nutritional support, to neurons. Normal astroglia function is necessary to maintain the BBB. Disruption of astrogliafunctions may lead to astrogliosis and inflammatory signaling in the CNS. Manganese may:

- decrease glutamine uptake by astroglia (in vitro)

- disrupt glucose synthesis by the astroglia

- inhibit the enzyme glutamine synthetase. Within astroglia

- decrease synthesis of tricarboxylic acid cycle intermediaries necessary for cellular energy production

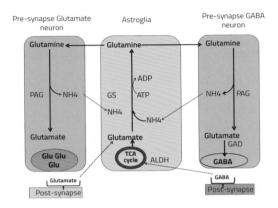

FIGURE 12.
Excitatory amino acid transporters (EAATs) are found on the astroglia and function to keep extracellular Glutamate levels low.

Legend: ALDH = succinate semialdehyde dehydrogenase; GAD = glutamate decarboxylase; Glu = glutamate in vesicle; GS = glutamine synthetase; PAG = phosphate activated glutaminase; TCA = tricarboxylic acid cycle. Wikimedia Commons image modified by Andrea Gruszecki.

Extracellular glutamate is regulated by a complex, unique network of release and reuptake mechanisms. Most of these mechanisms are rarely depicted in models of glutamate excitatory signaling. Extracellular glutamate releases occur due to cell membrane cystine-glutamate antiporter (system x_c^-) exchanges and volume-sensitive organic anion channels (sodium-dependent Glu transporters). Extracellular glutamate may alter activity by binding with extra-synaptic high-affinity glutamate receptors, including NMDA and metabotropic glutamate receptors (mGluRs). N-acetylcysteine upregulates antiporter system x_c^- in animal studies, but may be contraindicated in cases of congenital hypercystinuria. Studies in knockout mice indicate that a complete failure of system x_c^- may decrease extracelluar

glutamate in the CNS. Impairment of the glutamate recycling process facilitated by astroglia is considered a major contributing factor in neuropathology and is being researched as a causative factor in neurodegenerative diseases such as Alzheimer's, Parkinson's and amyotrophic lateral sclerosis (ALS).

In the periphery, current research suggests that enteric (gastrointestinal) glia may be important in glutamatergic signaling within the gut, and that neurotransmitter receptors on the gut mucosa and glial cells may respond to dietary glutamate and monosodium glutamate (MSG). The stimulation of glutamate receptors in the gut has been associated with regulation of digestive processes, the protection of the upper gastrointestinal tract from low pH conditions, and the stimulation of the afferent vagal nerve. Glutamate may be primarily oxidized and metabolized in the intestines, and serves to nourish the enterocytes of the gut mucosa as glutamine. Amino acid decarboxylation reactions in the gastrointestinal microbiota are known to generate biogenic amines and neuroactive molecules which may not only affect the levels of glutamate and GABA, but affect gut function. Animal studies indicate that free glutamate in the gut lumen may activate the vagus nerve and stimulate the brain. Glutamate signaling via taste and gut receptors may affect physiologic functions such as digestion, thermoregulation and energy production.

Receptors:

Glutamate signaling may occur through a variety of Glutamate receptors. There are four types of glutamate receptors. Combinations of different glutamate receptor subtypes may be found in different areas of the brain and the peripheral nervous system, and may determine how individual neurons respond to glutamate. Glutamate receptor function or conformation may be affected by mutations or single nucleotide polymorphisms (SNPs) in the DNA that codes for each receptor subtype.

Ionotropic receptors regulate sodium, potassium or calcium (charged ions) flow into and out of neurons. The level of ions inside the neuron determines its action potential and ability to fire. There are three families of ionotropic receptors:

Amino-3-hydroxy-5-methyl-4-isoxazole propionic acid (AMPA)

- control sodium and potassium influx into neurons

- post-synaptic

- mediate fast excitatory transmissions in the brain

- AMPA receptors have been found in the gastrointestinal tract (animal studies)

- GluR1-4 are AMPA receptors

Kainate receptors

- control sodium and potassium influx into neurons

- primarily pre-synaptic

- may regulate glutamate release

- GluR5-7 and GluR KA-1 and -2 are kainate receptors

N-methyl-D-aspartate (NMDA)

- controls calcium influx and sodium/potassium influx

  - binding of magnesium ions in the receptor's ion channel prevents the influx of calcium and acts as a receptor blocker

- dysfunctions may contribute to neuropsychiatric disorders (mood, schizophrenia)

- animal studies indicate that NMDA receptors may contribute to learning conditioned fear (fear-potential startle), which may contribute to development of post-traumatic stress disorder (PTSD)

- primarily post-synaptic

- receptors are concentrated in the limbic system of the brain

- NMDA receptors have been found in the gastrointestinal tract (animal studies)

- animal studies indicate that exercise may upregulate NMDA receptor expression

Multiple receptor subtypes

- NMDA R1 A-G and NMDA R2 A-D

Preclinical studies indicate that NMDA glutamatergic signaling may influence the formation of conditioned fear memories. Abnormal baseline and fear-potentiated startle symptoms have been observed in patients with post-traumatic stress disorder, suggesting that disturbed glutamate signaling may contribute to anxiety. Animal studies indicate that chronic stress down-regulates NMDA and AMPA receptor expression in the brain secondary to the stimulation of glucocorticoid receptors. The down-regulation of the glutamate receptors affected glutamate signaling and memory function in the experimental animals.

Metabotropic glutamate receptor (mGluRs) activity occurs primarily via second messenger signaling through cyclic adenosine monophosphate (cAMP) or phosphorylation of proteins. mGluRs are G-protein coupled receptors similar to dopamine, norepinephrine or serotonin receptors.

They are divided into three types:

Type I

- post-synaptic

- excitatory

- concentrated in amygdale, thalamus, hippocampus

- mGluR1 and mGluR5

Type II

- pre-synaptic glutamate release

- inhibitory

- mGluR2 and mGluR3

Type III

- primarily pre-synaptic (glutamate and GABA neurons)

- neuromodulators in brain

- mGluR 4 and mGluR 6-8

Some anxiety symptoms have been associated with changes in mGluRs. Metabolomic type III receptors are found in nerve pathways commonly overactive in Parkinson's disease. Animal studies indicate that metabolomic type I and II glutamate receptors may contribute to heart rate and blood pressure regulation.

Consider:

- Glutathione status (**Glutathione; erythrocytes**)

- Oxidative stress (**DNA Oxidative Damage Assay/8-OHdG**)

- Methionine metabolism and methylation pathways (**Plasma Methylation Profile, DNA Methylation Pathway**)

- Nutrient element (mineral) and manganese status (**RBC Elements**)

- Digestion and absorption (**Comprehensive Stool Analysis**)

References:

Akiba, Yasutada; Kaunitz, Jonathan D (2009)
Luminal chemosensing and upper gastrointestinal mucosal defenses
Am J Clin Nutr vol. 90 (3) p. 826S-831

Bridges, Richard; Lutgen, Victoria; Lobner, Doug; Baker, David A (2012)
Thinking outside the cleft to understand synaptic activity: contribution of the cystine-glutamate antiporter (System xc-) to normal and pathological glutamatergic signaling.

Pharmacological reviews vol. 64 (3) p. 780-802

Burrin, Douglas G; Stoll, Barbara (2009)
Metabolic fate and function of dietary glutamate in the gut
Am J Clin Nutr vol. 90 (3) p. 850S-856

Cotman, Carl W.; Kahle, Jennifer S.; Miller, Stephan E.; Ulas, Jolanta and Bridges, Richard J. (2000)
Excitatory Amino Acid Neurotransmission
Neuropsychopharmacology – 5th Generation of Progress
Lippincott, Williams, & Wilkins, Philadelphia, Pennsylvania, 2002

Dai, Zhao-Lai; Wu, Guoyao; Zhu, Wei-Yun (2011)
Amino acid metabolism in intestinal bacteria: links between gut ecology and host health
Frontiers in Bioscience 16, 1768-1786, January 1, 2011

De Bundel, Dimitri; Schallier, Anneleen; Loyens, Ellen; Fernando, Ruani; Miyashita, Hirohisa et al. (2011)
J. Neurosci. vol. 31 (15) p. 5792-5803
Loss of System xFormula Does Not Induce Oxidative Stress But Decreases Extracellular Glutamate in Hippocampus and Influences Spatial Working Memory and Limbic Seizure Susceptibility

Julio-Pieper, Marcela; Flor, Peter J.; Dinan, Timothy G. and Cryan, John F. (2011)
PHARMACOLOGICAL REVIEWS Vol. 63, No. 1
Pharmacol Rev 63:35–58, 2011

Kondoh, Takashi; Mallick, Hruda Nanda; Torii, Kunio (2009)
Activation of the gut-brain axis by dietary glutamate and physiologic significance in energy homeostasis
Am J Clin Nutr vol. 90 (3) p. 832S-837

Labow, Brian I.; Souba, Wiley W.; Abcouwer, Steve F. (2001)
Mechanisms Governing the Expression of the Enzymes of Glutamine Metabolism-- Glutaminase and Glutamine Synthetase
J. Nutr. vol. 131 (9) p. 2467S-2474

Li, X C; Beart, P M; Monn, J A; Jones, N M; Widdop, R E (1999)
Type I and II metabotropic glutamate receptor agonists and antagonists evoke cardiovascular effects after intrathecal administration in conscious rats.
British journal of pharmacology vol. 128 (3) p. 823-9

H T Liu, Markus W. Hollmann (2001)
Modulation of NMDA receptor function by ketamine and magnesium: Part I.
Anesthesia and analgesia vol. 92 (5) p. 1173 - 81

Park, Joon-Ki; Lee, Sam-Jun; Kim, Tae-Won (2014)
Treadmill exercise enhances NMDA receptor expression in schizophrenia mice.
Journal of exercise rehabilitation vol. 10 (1) p.

Torii, Kunio; Uneyama, Hisayuki; Nakamura, Eiji (2013)
Physiological roles of dietary glutamate signaling via gut-brain axis due to efficient digestion and absorption.
Journal of gastroenterology vol. 48 (4) p. 442-51

Tsapakis, Eva M.; Travis, Michael J. (2002)
Glutamate and psychiatric disorders
Adv. Psychiatr. Treat. vol. 8 (3) p. 189-197

Valentine, Gerald W; Sanacora, Gerard (2009)
Targeting glial physiology and glutamate cycling in the treatment of depression.
Biochemical pharmacology vol. 78 (5) p. 431-9

Willard, Stacey S.; Koochekpour, Shahriar. (2013)
Glutamate, Glutamate Receptors, and Downstream Signaling Pathways.
Int J Biol Sci 2013; 9(9):948-959. doi:10.7150/ijbs.6426

Yuen, Eunice Y.; Wei, Jing; Liu, Wenhua; Zhong, Ping; Li, Xiangning et al. (2012) Repeated Stress Causes Cognitive Impairment by Suppressing Glutamate Receptor Expression and Function in Prefrontal Cortex *Neuron* vol. 73 (5) p. 962-977

Gamma-aminobutyric acid (GABA)

Gamma-aminobutyric acid (GABA) functions as an inhibitory neurotransmitter in the central nervous system (CNS). GABA acts in opposition to glutamate, the primary excitatory neurotransmitter. Studies demonstrate decreased GABA levels in animal models of depression, and clinical studies report low plasma and cerebro-spinal fluid GABA levels in mood disorder patients. Very recent evidence indicates that GABA-mediated signals may contribute to synchronized neural network oscillations in the brain that facilitate cognition and information processing. Disruption of GABA transmission at synapses may perturb the neural oscillations and may contribute to symptoms of schizophrenia.

GABA and dopamine "crosstalk" is modulated by glutamate and creates a complex interaction between these neurotransmitters and their effects. GABA may, through GABA receptor activity, induce norepinephrine activity in the brain (animal studies), even as GABA may be affected by the activity of adrenergic receptors. GABA may modulate serotonin signaling in certain areas of the brain, and GABA may respond to signals from 5-HT serotonin receptors. Disruptions in GABA signaling during development affects nerve cell migration, maturation and differentiation; GABA signaling is mostly excitatory during early development. Altered

GABA signaling has been associated with neurodevelopmental disorders such as autism, Fragile X, Down's syndrome, schizophrenia, Tourette's syndrome and neurofibromatosis. Adult neuron generation and post-development neural plasticity is also regulated by GABA signaling. Astroglia possesses GABA receptors; they may be sensitive to, and release, GABA.

GABA is found throughout the gastrointestinal tract (GIT), where it may both serve as a neurotransmitter and mediate endocrine responses. Myenteric neurons in the gut regulate motility; 5-8% of myenteric neurons contain GABA. GABA-B receptors contribute to the regulation of gastric emptying, stomach pH and gut motility. GABA transporters are found in cells of the enteric (GIT) nervous system that innervate the small intestine (duodenum, ileum) and the large intestine. In vitro and animal studies indicate that GABA signaling may also affect intestinal fluid levels, electrolyte levels, serotonin release and nitric oxide signaling in the gut.

The GABA signaling system is affected by ethanol (alcohol) and ingestion has been associated with some of the symptoms associated with drinking such as poor coordination sedation, loss of inhibition, and withdrawal.

Effects:

Decreased GABA levels have been associated with neurological disorders such as Huntington's chorea, Parkinson's and Alzheimer's disease. GABA deficiency may also play a role in psychiatric disorders such as anxiety, depression, chronic pain, panic, or mania. Studies indicate that plasma GABA levels are lower in 40% of depressed, manic or euthymic (neither manic nor depressed) bipolar patients, and that the low plasma levels persist even after treatment or recovery. Other studies indicate that plasma GABA levels were not correlated with severity of depression in the study subjects; however additional research indicates that association of low GABA levels and mood disorder may be familial. Low plasma GABA levels have been associated with mood disorders in children and adolescents. Low plasma GABA levels have also been associated with premenstrual dysphoric disorder. GABA deficiency has not been directly associated with epilepsy, but disorders of GABA receptors have been.

Excess urinary GABA may occur due to nutritional deficiency or bacterial overgrowth. GABA, and other amino acids that require B-6 dependent transamination (leucine, isoleucine, valine) may be elevated due to vitamin B-6 deficiency. GABA may be artifactually elevated during bacterial urinary tract infections or, occasionally, due to gastrointestinal infections (dysbiosis). GABA may be produced or metabolized by gastrointestinal bacteria, including *Lactobacilli* and *Bifidobacteria*. The monoamine oxidase inhibitor phenelzine may increase GABA levels (animal study). Hyperforin, one of the active ingredients in Hypericum (St John's wort) extract may elevate GABA levels (animal studies). Magnetic resonance imaging studies

have measured elevated GABA levels in the brain cortex of primary insomniacs.

The known genetic disorders of GABA metabolism are succinic semialdehyde dehydrogenase (SSADH) deficiency, GABA-transaminase deficiency, and homocarnosinosis. All present early in life with a variety of neurological symptoms. GABA-transaminase deficiency, and homocarnosinosis are extremely rare and require specialized testing for diagnosis. The mutation causing SSADH deficiency is also rare, but many single nucleotide polymorphisms (SNPs) for this enzyme have been discovered; research continues to determine what, if any, functional effects the SNPs may have; SSADH may be inhibited by oxidative stress. True SSADH deficiency presents with elevated urine gamma-hydroxybutyric acid (GHB) and a constellation of neuropsychiatric signs, including developmental delay, mental retardation, language deficit, hypotonia, cerebellar ataxia, hyporeflexia, sleep disturbances, aggression, obsessive–compulsive disorder, inattention and hyperactivity. Epilepsy affects approximately half of these patients and is usually generalized. Taurine is considered a GABA-A receptor agonist and has been used (up to 3 grams daily) with success in some patients with SSADH deficiency, although the mechanism of action remains unclear.

Synthesis and Metabolism:

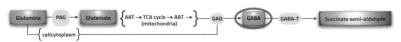

GABA is synthesized from glutamate by L-glutamate decarboxylase (GAD). GAD is expressed in GABA-ergic neurons in the CNS and requires a pyridoxal-5'-phosphate (B6) cofactor. GAD has two isoforms in the adult and two additional isoforms are expressed during early development. GAD67 synthesizes GABA in the body of the neuron. GAD65 is located in the axon terminals near the nerve synapse, and provides additional GABA as needed to meet the functional demands of neuron activity. GAD67 expression is controlled by the gene GAD1; GAD65 expression is controlled by GAD2, a gene on a separate chromosome. Early evidence from a human twin study indicates that some GAD1 haplotypes (gene groupings) may be associated with increased risk of neuropsychiatric disorders. The study found no such association for GAD2 haplotypes. Animal studies associate GAD function and behavior; the studies indicate that even subtle decreases in GABA signaling may alter behavior. Recently, a link has been made between GAD deficiency and nonsyndromic cleft lip or cleft palate.

GABA synthesis occurs in the cytosol, and GABA is transported into synaptic vesicles for storage by vesicular GABA transporters (vGATs). Lithium may increase GAD activity (animal studies). Once released, GABA is removed from the neural synapse through active transport back into the vesicles. GABA re-uptake requires dedicated transmembrane transporters. In the CNS, GABA uptake primarily occurs through the activity of the plasma membrane GABA transporter 1 (GAT1) which takes up GABA through neuron and glial membranes. GAT1 activity may be inhibited by nitric oxide. A second GABA transporter, GAT2, is found in the gastrointestinal tract, and GAT3 is expressed in adult astroglia. Any GABA that remains in the synapse is taken up by astroglia and metabolized by GABA transaminases (GABA-T), a group of three enzymes that breaks GABA down (using various

substrates) into succinic semialdehyde, glutamate and either glycine or alanine. Succinic semialdehyde is then converted into succinate by SSADH in the mitochondria for use in the tri-carboxylic acid (TCA) cycle.

Amino acid decarboxylation reactions in the gastrointestinal microbiota are known to generate neuroactive molecules which may not only contribute to the levels of glutamate and GABA, but affect gut function. GAD is also expressed peripherally in pancreatic B-cells, which are known to produce GABA. GABA neurons are known to innervate the pancreas. In vitro studies indicate that GAD65 may act as an autoantigen, and may play a role in the development of diabetes. Research continues into the function of GABA in the pancreas.

Receptors:

GABA receptors are found throughout the brain. There are two primary groups of GABA receptors, GABA-A receptors are ionotropic, GABA-B receptors are metabotropic. Animal studies indicate that chronic administration of antidepressants (such as phenelzine and imipramine), benzodiazepines (such as alprazolam, lorazepam, and diazepam), and mood stabilizers (such as lamotrigine) may differentially modulate the gene expression of GABA receptor subunits, particularly for GABA-A receptors. GABA receptor functions may affect blood sugar levels and insulin responses.

GABA-A receptors

Dysfunction of GABA-A receptor subunits may affect memory, learning, moods, fatigue, sedation level, stress-induced depression, coordination, balance, seizures, eating and alcohol use behaviors. Chronic administration of anti-depressant medications may decrease the expression of GABA-A receptors in the brain (animal studies). GABA-A receptors:

- Are directly affected by ethanol, which functions as a receptor agonist

- Function by allowing chloride influx through cell membranes into nerve cells (action potential)

- May be in the synapse or extrasynaptic

- Receptor subtypes α, β, γ, δ, ϵ – each subtype and its subunits may bind to different types of molecules – in addition to GABA, many bind to sedative drugs (barbiturates), anxiolytics (benzo-diazepines), anesthetics and ethanol

- β-adrenergic receptor signaling (norepinephrine, epinephrine) signaling may affect GABA receptor function through second messenger signaling (increased phosphorylation of GABA receptors) and enhance GABA-A receptor activity

- Metabolites of progesterone, testosterone, and stress hormone deoxycorticosterone may act as GABA-A receptor agonists (in vitro studies)

- Dehydroepiandrosterone sulfate (DHEA-S), pregnenolone sulfate (and similar 3-betahydroxy-pregnane steroids) may antagonize GABA-A receptors (in vitro studies)

- May be modulated by zinc; in vitro studies have shown that zinc antagonizes GABA neuron functions

- Activation of GABA-A receptors in the pancreas decreases insulin and glucagon excretion (in vitro)

GABA-B receptors

Abnormal regulation of GABA-B receptor activity may contribute to mood disorders, visceral pain perception and affect digestive functions.

- Altered activity has been associated with several neuropsychiatric disorders

- Found on excitatory and inhibitory neurons; contribute to the function of multi-neuron "circuits"

- Inhibit multiple glutamate vesicle releases from pre-synaptic terminals (decrease synaptic glutamate signaling)

- Two metabotropic isoforms act to regulate potassium influx into neurons by second-messenger signaling (action potential)

- Inhibit calcium permeability of NMDA receptors to inhibit calcium-dependent signaling ins post-synaptic neurons (action potential)

- Valproate, lithium and carbamazepine may upregulate GABA-B receptors (animal studies)

- Activation of GABA-B receptors in the pancreas increases insulin release (in vitro)

- Contribute to spinal and vagal afferent (from periphery to CNS) signaling and may affect visceral pain (nociception) perception by decreasing afferent signaling and enhancing anti-nociceptive signaling

- Are abundant in the gastrointestinal (GI) and may contribute to gastric emptying, gastric pH, gut motility, intestinal fluid levels, electrolyte levels, serotonin release and nitric oxide signaling in the gut.

Endozepines are nonbenzodiazepine, nonprotein molecules produced within the body. In vitro studies indicate that endozepines secreted from astroglia may bind to GABA-A receptors and act like benzodiazepines on the receptors. GABA signaling may also be modified by the activity of the diazepam binding inhibitor (DBI), a protein which may displace endozepines and benzodiazepines from GABA-A receptor binding sites (in vitro studies).

Consider:

- Assess dysbiosis (**Comprehensive Stool Analysis**)

- Zinc status (**RBC Elements**)

- Calcium and potassium status (**Serum Elements**)

References:

Brambilla, P; Perez, J; Barale, F; Schettini, G; Soares, J C (2003)
GABAergic dysfunction in mood disorders
Nature Publishing Group vol. 8 (8) p. 721-737

Chalifoux, Jason R; Carter, Adam G (2011)
GABAB receptor modulation of synaptic function.
Current opinion in neurobiology vol. 21 (2) p. 339-44

Christian, Catherine A.; Huguenard, John R. (2013)
Astrocytes potentiate GABAergic transmission in the thalamic reticular nucleus via endozepine signaling
PNAS vol. 110 (50) p. 20278-20283

Claus, Sandrine P; Tsang, Tsz M; Wang, Yulan; Cloarec, Olivier; Skordi, Eleni et al. (2008)
Systemic multicompartmental effects of the gut microbiome on mouse metabolic phenotypes.
Molecular Systems Biology vol. 4 (1) p. 219

Davies, Martin (2003)
The role of GABAA receptors in mediating the effects of alcohol in the central nervous system.
Journal of psychiatry & neuroscience : JPN vol. 28 (4) p. 263-74

Neuropsychopharmacology: The Fifth Generation of Progress
Davis, et al.
Lippincott, Williams, & Wilkins, Philadelphia, Pennsylvania, 2002

Gajcy, K.; Lochynski, S.; Librowski, T (2010)
A Role of GABA Analogues in the Treatment of Neurological Diseases
Current Medicinal Chemistry, Volume 17, Number 22, August 2010, pp. 2338-2347(10)

Gonzalez-Burgos, Guillermo; Fish, Kenneth N; Lewis, David A (2011)
GABA neuron alterations, cortical circuit dysfunction and cognitive deficits in schizophrenia.
Neural plasticity vol. 2011 p. 723184

Hettema, J M; An, S S; Neale, M C; Bukszar, J; van den Oord, E J C G et al. (2006)
Association between glutamic acid decarboxylase genes and anxiety disorders, major depression, and neuroticism.
Molecular psychiatry vol. 11 (8) p. 752-62

Hyland, Niall P; Cryan, John F (2010)
A Gut Feeling about GABA: Focus on GABA(B) Receptors.
Frontiers in pharmacology vol. 1 p. 124

Jayakrishnan, Bindu; Hoke, David E; Langendorf, Christopher G; Buckle, Ashley M; Rowley, Merrill J (2011)
An analysis of the cross-reactivity of autoantibodies to GAD65 and GAD67 in diabetes.
PloS one vol. 6 (4) p. e18411

Kim, Kyung-Jin; Pearl, Phillip L; Jensen, Kimmo; Snead, O Carter; Malaspina, Patrizia et al. (2011)
Succinic semialdehyde dehydrogenase: biochemical-molecular-clinical disease

mechanisms, redox regulation, and functional significance.
Antioxidants & redox signaling vol. 15 (3) p. 691-718

Online Mendelian Inheritance in Man (OMIM)
Diazepam binding inhibitor; DBI
Accessed 26 December 2014
Pearl, Phillip L; Hartka, Thomas R; Cabalza, Jessica L; Taylor, Jacob; Gibson, Michael K (2006)
Inherited disorders of GABA metabolism.
Future neurology vol. 1 (5) p. 631-636

Taneera, J; Jin, Z; Jin, Y; Muhammed, S J; Zhang, E et al. (2012)
-Aminobutyric acid (GABA) signalling in human pancreatic islets is altered in type 2 diabetes.
Diabetologia vol. 55 (7) p. 1985-94

Wang, Mingde (2011)
Neurosteroids and GABA-A Receptor Function.
Frontiers in endocrinology vol. 2 p. 44

Tyrosine

Tyrosine is a non-essential amino acid that may be acquired from dietary proteins or synthesized from dietary phenylalanine, an essential amino acid. Tyrosine is the precursor for the catecholamine neurotransmitters dopamine, norepinephrine and epinephrine; tyrosine availability may affect the synthesis of these catecholamines. Tyrosine is also the precursor for thyroxine (thyroid hormone) and melanin (skin pigment). The proportion of dietary tyrosine that enters systemic circulation from the diet is controlled by the enzyme tyrosine aminotransferase (TAT) in liver and kidney. Tyrosine may be considered a conditionally essential amino acid if its precursor phenylalanine is deficient or in patients with phenylketonuria (PKU),

an inherited disorder of phenylalanine metabolism.

Effects:

Decreased tyrosine levels may impair both spatial recognition memory and mental performance. Low tyrosine levels may increase irritability scores during psychological challenge testing. Human studies of short-term dietary tyrosine depletion indicate that low tyrosine levels may increase prolactin hormone levels and may lower mood and energy levels. Tyrosine depletion has also been reported to decrease observational clinical ratings for manic symptoms in patients. Long-term depletion of dietary tyrosine may result in catecholamine neurotransmitter depletion, which may affect mood. Low tyrosine levels have been associated with decreases in body temperature and thyroid function. Elevated glucocorticoid, insulin, glucagon, or tryptophan levels may induce liver tyrosine aminotransferase (TAT), which may decrease tyrosine levels. Conversion of phenylalanine to tyrosine requires tetrahydrobiopterin (BH4). Tyrosine levels may decrease if phenylalanine is deficient or in patients with PKU. Human studies indicate that Tyrosine supplementation may improve cognition and performance under stressful conditions.

Excess tyrosine levels may occur due to heritable enzyme defects, liver disease, or supplementation. Elevated tyrosine levels may interfere with medications such as monoamine oxidase inhibitors (MAOIs), thyroid hormone replacement and L-dopa replacement. Migraine headaches and hyperthyroid conditions may be exacerbated by elevated tyrosine levels. High levels of tyrosine may result in elevated levels of the trace amine tyramine.

A decrease in the activity of tyrosine hydroxylase (TH), which metabolizes tyrosine to L-3,4-dihydroxyphenylalanine (L-DOPA), may elevate tyrosine levels and decrease levels of dopamine and norepinephrine. TH requires iron and tetrahydrobiopterin (BH4) cofactors. Mutation of tyrosine aminotransferase (TAT) may elevate tyrosine levels in plasma and urine (type II tyrosinemia); it is possible that single nucleotide polymorphisms (SNPs) may also alter TAT activity, research continues in this area. TAT requires pyridoxal phosphate (B6) and alpha-ketoglutarate as cofactors and oxidative stress has been shown to lower TAT activity (in vitro).

Elevated plasma tyrosine levels have been associated with seizures or developmental delays. Tyrosine hydroxylase (TH) deficiency is a group of rare inherited disorders that presents early in life in one of three forms:

- dystonia

  - mildest form with onset from 1-6 years; usually presents with lower limb dystonia (involuntary muscle contractions) or difficulty walking, symptoms may worsen in the evening and improve in morning after sleep
  - infantile Parkinsonism with motor delays
  - severe form with onset from 3-12 months; motor milestones are delayed, presents with truncal hypotonia and Parkinson's symptoms

- progressive infantile encephalopathy

  - most severe form with onset before 6 months; presents with delay in motor development, truncal hypotonia, limb hypertonia (rigid/spastic) hyperreflexia, ptosis, intellectual disability, lethargy (with sweating and drooling) alternates with irritability

Synthesis and metabolism:

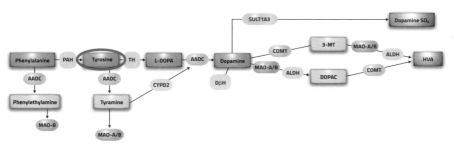

Phenylalanine, an essential amino acid is converted into tyrosine via the enzyme phenylalanine hydroxylase; the enzyme requires a tetrahydrobiopterin (BH4) cofactor. Tyrosine is then converted into L-DOPA by tyrosine hydroxylase (TH), which requires BH4 and an iron cofactor. Tyrosine hydroxylase is located in dopamine and norepinephrine neurons in various brain areas. In the pe-

riphery, TH is found in the adrenal medulla and in sympathetic ganglia (nerve clusters). Animal studies indicate that selenium deficient diets increase the activity of tyrosine hydroxylase two-fold.

Selenium deficiency also decreased the expression of glutathione peroxidase and glutathione reductase; decreased expression of these enzymes may increase intracellular oxidative stress. TH enzyme function may be down-regulated by oxidative stress, nitrosative stress and thiolation (reactions with sulfur amino acids). Single nucleotide polymorphisms (SNPs) in the genes coding for tyrosine hydroxylase have been associated with altered stress responses, blood pressure, heart rate and norepinephrine secretion. Evidence that TH polymorphisms contribute to neuropsychiatric disorders remains contradictory.

Levels of Tyrosine in the brain may be influenced by the plasma levels of other amino acids, as several amino acids may compete for a single transporter across the blood brain barrier (BBB). Brain tyrosine levels control the rate of synthesis for the catecholamine neurotransmitters in the central nervous system (CNS). Tyrosine is metabolized to glutamate by tyrosine aminotransferase (TAT), primarily in the liver.

Receptors:

There are no known receptors for the amino acid tyrosine.

Consider:

- Phenylalanine precursor status (**Amino Acids, Comprehensive Stool Analysis**)

- Selenium status (**RBC Elements**)

- Glutathione status (**Glutathione; erythrocytes**)

- Oxidative stress (**DNA Oxidative Damage Assay/8-OHdG**)

References:

Cansev, M.; Wurtman, R.J. (2007) Chapter 4
Aromatic Amino Acids in the Brain
Handbook of Neurochemistry and Molecular
Neurobiology
Springer US

Fernstrom, John D (2000)
Can nutrient supplements modify brain
function?
Am J Clin Nutr vol. 71 (6) p. 1669S-1673

Fernstrom, John D.; Fernstrom, Madelyn H.
(2007)
Tyrosine, Phenylalanine, and Catecholamine
Synthesis and Function in the Brain
J. Nutr. vol. 137 (6) p. 1539S-1547

Leyton, M; Young, SN; Pihl, RO; Etezadi, S;
Lauze, C et al. (2000)
Effects on Mood of Acute Phenylalanine/
Tyrosine Depletion in Healthy Women
*American College of
Neuropsychopharmacology* vol. 22 (1) p.
52-63

Matthews, Dwight E. (2007)
An Overview of Phenylalanine and Tyrosine
Kinetics in Humans
J. Nutr. vol. 137 (6) p. 1549S-1555

Rao, Fangwen; Zhang, Lian; Wessel, Jennifer;
Zhang, Kuixing; Wen, Gen et al. (2007)
Tyrosine Hydroxylase, the Rate-Limiting
Enzyme in Catecholamine Biosynthesis:
Discovery of Common Human Genetic
Variants Governing Transcription,
Autonomic Activity, and Blood Pressure
In Vivo
Circulation vol. 116 (9) p. 993-1006

Zhang, Lian; Rao, Fangwen; Wessel, Jennifer;
Kennedy, Brian P.; Rana, Brinda K. et al.
(2004)
Functional allelic heterogeneity and pleiotropy of a repeat polymorphism in tyrosine
hydroxylase: prediction of catecholamines and response to stress in twins
Physiol Genomics vol. 19 (3) p. 277-291

Tyramine

Tyramine is a trace amine derived from the essential amino acid phenylalanine. Trace amines are not considered neurotransmitters, they are believed to act as neuromodulators. The interaction of trace amines, and their receptors, in the brain may play a role in psychiatric and neurological disease processes. Experimental evidence suggests that dysregulation of trace amines may alter the levels of dopamine, norepinephrine or serotonin, and thereby contribute to neuropsychiatric disorders such as attention deficit hyperactivity disorder (ADHD), schizophrenia, depression and neurodegenerative diseases. Tyramine may potentiate neuron responses to dopamine and norepinephrine. *In vitro* and *in vivo* studies indicate that tyramine and phenylethylamine (PEA) may enhance neuron response to norepinephrine and dopamine signaling and may decrease post-synaptic responses to GABA-B receptor signaling. As a neuromodulator, evidence indicates that tyramine may also alter neuron responsiveness to monoamine neurotransmitters such as histamine and serotonin. Tyramine has been shown to inhibit the responses of gamma-aminobutyric acid (GABA) receptors in vitro and both in vitro and in vivo studies indicate that tyramine may inhibit prolactin secretion. Trace amines may also alter neuron active transport mechanisms and vesicle dynamics. Clinically, trace amines are generally considered sympathomimetic (they mimic the action of sympathetic nerve stimulation), they may affect vasoconstriction and blood pressure. In large, supra-physiologic doses, the effects of trace amines are similar to amphetamines.

Effects:

Decreased levels of tyramine or deficient trace amine functions may contribute to some depressive disorders. Altered aromatic L-amino acid decarboxylase (AADC) activity may alter trace amine levels which may affect dopamine signaling. Activation of monoamine neurotransmitter receptors (via receptor agonists or electrical stimulation) decreases AADC activity and trace amine levels. Loss of D-neurons containing AADC has been associated with some forms of schizophrenia. Reserpine may deplete CNS levels of trace amines.

Excess tyramine and increased AADC activity have been associated with some forms of schizophrenia, and may resemble the effects of amphetamines: increased alertness, irritability, euphoria, insomnia, tachycardia, tremor, decreased appetite and changes in blood pressure. Nausea, vomiting, shortness of breath, sweating, increased body temperature, and headache have also been reported. Excess tryamine in the kidney may increase urine output. Increased AADC activity may increase trace amine levels without affecting the levels of monoamine neurotransmitters. Decreased monoamine neurotransmitter receptor activation (receptor antagonists, neurotransmitter depletion) may result in an increase in AADC activity and increased trace amine levels. Elevated plasma and urinary tyramine levels have been reported in Reye's Syndrome.

Elevated tyramine levels do not seem to correlate with migraine or cluster headaches in research, but elevated levels of the tyramine metabolite octopamine have been associated with migraine and cluster headaches. Tyramine and other sympathomimetic amines, promote the release of norepinephrine from nerve endings. Foodstuffs such as hard cheeses and red wines contain large amounts of tyramine. Normally, dietary tyramine is metabolized in the gastrointestinal tract and liver before the amine can enter the systemic circulation. If monoamine oxidase A (MAO-A) is inhibited by medication or if enzyme function is deficient, tyramine is able to reach the sympathetic nerve terminals, and paroxysmal hypertension and headache may result from release of vesicular norepinephrine.

Trace amines may be generated in the gastrointestinal tract by protein-fermenting gut bacteria after a protein-rich meal, and they may be found in a variety of foods as the result of food spoilage or deliberate fermentation. Dietary trace amines are usually metabolized quickly by MAO enzymes. Elevated levels of trace amines may occur due to phenylketonuria, ergot poisoning or the use of monoamine oxidase inhibitors (MAOIs). Elevated levels of the precursor amino acid tyrosine may result in elevated levels of tyramine.

Synthesis and Metabolism:

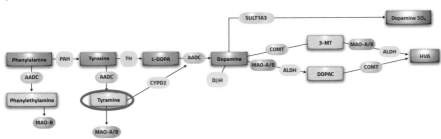

Tyramine is the metabolite of the aromatic amino acid tyrosine. It is synthesized by aromatic L-amino acid decarboxylase (AADC), which is the rate-limiting step for trace amine synthesis. AADC is widely expressed within the CNS and throughout the body, and requires pyridoxal phosphate (vitamin B6) as a cofactor. Trace amines may also be synthesized through the metabolism of secondary amines (molecules that contain N-methyltyramine). Tyramine, and other trace amines are found at low (nanomolar) levels in the brain and the peripheral nervous system; they represent less than 1% of the total volume of biogenic amines in the central nervous system (CNS). Secondary amines may be converted to trace amines by methyltransferase enzymes, which are

also widely expressed in the brain and peripheral tissues. Methyltransferase enzymes require S-adnosylmethionine (SAM) as a cofactor. SAM must be synthesized inside neurons behind the blood brain barrier through an enzyme pathway now commonly referred to as the methylation cycle.

In vitro and animal studies indicate that the cytochrome P450 enzyme CYP2D may, in the brain, convert tyramine into dopamine. The contribution of this pathway to the dopamine pool, and its effects on neurotransmitter and trace amine homeostasis, are still under investigation. CYP2D expression may be upregulated by nicotine, alcohol and some psycho-active drugs (such as nefazodone and clozapine). CYP2D expression may be inhibited by antidepressant medications.

Tyramine is metabolized by both the A and B forms of monoamine oxidase (MAO). Animal studies indicate that the addition of selenium and tocopherols to the diet may increase antioxidant capacity and decrease MAO-B activity. With the exception of PEA, trace amines are considered short-acting and have a half-life of less than thirty seconds. Tyramine may be stored in synaptic vesicles; research continues in this area. Most trace amines are not stored, but disperse by diffusion through cell membranes. Trace amines and their metabolites are excreted by the kidney in urine.

Receptors:

The trace amine-associated receptors (TAARs) are a recently discovered class of receptors that respond to various trace amines. Most TAARs activity is the result of second messenger signaling through cyclic adenosine monophosphate (cAMP) and protein phosphorylation. TAARs are found in the CNS and in the periphery are primarily found in the gastrointestinal tract, lung, and kidneys. In other mammals, some TAARs may serve as olfactory chemoreceptors and may respond to stimulation by odorous amines. Research continues into the function of TAARs and their ligands as not all TAAR subtypes respond to known trace amines. Mutations or single nucleotide polymorphisms in the nine genes coding for TAARs may affect receptor conformation or function, which may increase susceptibility risk for schizophrenia or bipolar disorders. In vitro and in vivo studies indicate:

- TAAR1
  - Intracellular expression

  - Binds to tyramine and PEA with greatest affinity
  - May modulate catecholamines and serotonin by altering cell membrane transport or receptor function
  - Expressed in the CNS and in leukocytes, gastrointestinal tract, lung, and kidneys
    - has been shown in vitro to assist leukocyte chemotaxis towards trace amines; binding of trace amines to TAAR1 in leukocytes has been shown in vitro to promote cytokine release
  - Binds with amphetamines and psychotropic agents (ergot alkaloids, bromocriptine, lisuride, D-lysergic acid diethylamide (LSD), 3,4-methylenedioxy-methamphetamine [MDMA or ecstasy])
  - Interacts with the thyroid hormone derivative 3-iodothyronamines, which may affect temperature regulation and cardiac contractility (in vivo)

- TAAR2
  - Has been shown in vitro to assist leukocyte chemotaxis towards trace amines; binding of trace amines to TAAR2 in leukocytes has been shown in vitro to promote cytokine release
  - Nonsense mutation may contribute to some cases of schizophrenia

- TAAR5
  - Function in humans unknown

- TAAR6
  - Expressed in the amygdala of the brain and in leukocytes, kidneys

- SNP has been associated with increased familial susceptibility to schizophrenia in those of European or African-American ancestry

- TAAR8

  - Expressed in the amygdala of the brain and in leukocytes, kidneys

- TAAR9

  - Expressed in pituitary and in leukocytes, kidney and skeletal muscle

Trace amines may activate sigma receptors and modulate potassium and calcium channels (in vitro); altering the level of ions inside neurons may change their action potential and firing rate.

Consider:

- Selenium status (**RBC Elements**)

- Glutathione status (**Glutathione; erythrocytes**)

- Oxidative stress (**DNA Oxidative Damage Assay/8-OHdG**)

- Methylation pathway activity (**Plasma Methylation Profile, DNA Methylation Pathway**)

References:

Berry, M.D. (2007)
The Potential of Trace Amines and Their Receptors for Treating Neurological and Psychiatric Diseases
Reviews on Recent Clinical Trials, 2007, 2, 3-19

Berry, Mark D. (2004)
Mammalian central nervous system trace amines. Pharmacologic amphetamines, physiologic neuromodulators.
Journal of Neurochemistry, Volume 90, Issue 2, pages 257–271, July 2004

Goldstein, David S. (2008)
Genotype and Vascular Phenotype Linked by Catecholamine Systems
Circulation vol. 117 (4) p. 458-461

Haduch, Anna; Bromek, Ewa; Daniel, Władysława A (2013)
Role of brain cytochrome P450 (CYP2D) in the metabolism of monoaminergic neurotransmitters.
Pharmacological reports : PR vol. 65 (6) p. 1519-28

Ledonne, Ada; Berretta, Nicola; Davoli, Alessandro; Rizzo, Giada Ricciardo; Bernardi, Giorgio et al. (2011)
Electrophysiological effects of trace amines on mesencephalic dopaminergic neurons.
Frontiers in systems neuroscience vol. 5 p. 56

Miller, Gregory M (2011)
The emerging role of trace amine-associated receptor 1 in the functional regulation of monoamine transporters and dopaminergic activity.
Journal of neurochemistry vol. 116 (2) p. 164-76

Narang, Deepak; Tomlinson, Sara; Holt, Andrew; Darrell D. Mousseau, Glen B. Baker, DSc, FCAHS (2011)
Trace amines and their relevance to psychiatry and neurology: a brief overview
Bulletin of Clinical Psychopharmacology vol. 21 (1) p. 73-79

Goldstein, David S. (2008)
Genotype and Vascular Phenotype Linked by Catecholamine Systems
Circulation vol. 117 (4) p. 458-461

Zucchi, R; Chiellini, G; Scanlan, T S; Grandy, D K (2006)
Trace amine-associated receptors and their ligands.
British journal of pharmacology vol. 149 (8) p. 967-78

Phenylethylamine (PEA)

Phenylethylamine (B-phenylethylamine or PEA) is one of several trace amines present in the central nervous system at low (nanomolar) concentrations. The interaction of trace amines, and their receptors, in the brain may play a role in psychiatric and neurological disease processes. Experimental evidence suggests that dysregulation of trace amines may alter levels of dopamine, norepinephrine or serotonin, and thereby contribute to neuropsychiatric disorders such as attention deficit hyperactivity disorder (ADHD), schizophrenia, depression and neurodegenerative diseases. PEA may potentiate neuron responses to dopamine and norepinephrine. PEA excretion may be influenced by diurnal rhythms; larger amounts are excreted during the late evening and early morning hours. Clinically, trace amines are generally considered sympathomimetic (they mimic the action of sympathetic nerve stimulation), they may affect vasoconstriction and blood pressure. In large, supra-physiologic doses, the effects of trace amines are similar to amphetamines.

Effects:

Decreased PEA levels have been associated with Parkinson's disease, depression, attention deficit hyperactivity disorder (ADHD) and autism. In studies of ADHD patients, low levels of the precursor amino acid phenylalanine or decreased activity of aromatic L-amino acid decarboxylase (AADC), the enzyme that converts phenylalanine into PEA, may decrease PEA levels. AADC requires pyridoxal phosphate (vitamin B6) as a cofactor. Reserpine may deplete CNS levels of trace amines.

Excess PEA may occur due to supplementation. Elevated PEA levels have been reported during the use of monoamine oxidase inhibitors (MAOIs) or antipsychotic medications. Excess PEA may be the only clue to monoamine oxidase B (MAO-B) deficiency. Experiments in humans and animals associate PEA elevations with stress or anxiety. Elevations in PEA may contribute to anxiety disorders (animal studies). Very high levels may have amphetamine-like effects, and may induce seizures (animal studies). Patients with hypertension or bone disease may have elevated PEA levels. Exercise or high protein diets may also increase PEA levels. Inhibition of PEA catabolism (breakdown) has been associated with schizophrenia, as have elevated levels of PEA. Increased urinary excretion of PEA has been observed in paranoid schizophrenia.

PEA may be naturally occurring in plant foods, or may be incorporated into foods through deliberate bacterial fermentation. Trace amines may be generated in the gastrointestinal tract by protein-fermenting gut bacteria after a protein-rich meal, and they may be found in a variety of foods as the result of food spoilage or fermentation. Dietary trace amines are usually metabolized quickly by MAO enzymes. PEA is preferentially oxidized by MAO-B, and may be the only elevated urinary biomarker if MAOB is deficient. Dietary PEA is able to cross the blood brain barrier into the CNS. Elevated levels of trace amines may occur due to phenylketonuria (PKU), ergot poisoning or the use of medications such as MAO inhibitors (MAOIs).

Synthesis and Metabolism:

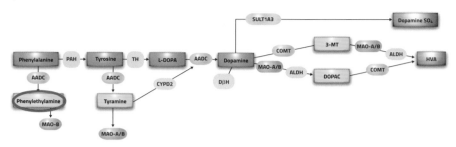

Trace amines derive from the aromatic amino acids (phenylalanine, tyrosine, tryptophan) through a decarboxylation reaction. This single-step process is catalyzed by aromatic L-amino acid decarboxylase (AADC), which requires pyridoxal phosphate (vitamin B6) as a cofactor. The action of AADC directly yields PEA from L-phenylalanine. AADC activity is dependent on dopamine levels, but not specific to dopamine signaling. AADC activity may be inhibited by autoimmune antibodies, or lack of precursor amino acids may affect PEA levels. PEA may not be stored; it crosses cell membranes easily and may act by local diffusion. Trace amines are metabolized by monoamine oxidase (MAO); PEA is primarily oxidized by MAO-B to to phenylacetic acid. Animal studies indicate that the addition of selenium and tocopherols to the diet increased antioxidant capacity and decreased MAO-B activity. Trace amines and their metabolites are excreted by the kidney in urine.

In vitro studies indicate that PEA may modulate dopamine, norepinephrine and serotonin monoamine transporters and reuptake mechanisms. PEA has been shown to depress gamma-aminobutyric acid (GABA)-B receptor-mediated responses in dopamine neurons (*in vitro*). PEA and tyramine may have endocrine effects and inhibit prolactin secretion (*in vitro* and *in vivo*). Animal studies indicate that PEA may increase adrenocorticotropic hormone (ACTH) and glucocorticoid levels. PEA has also been shown to stimulate acetylcholine release through activation of glutamate signaling pathways (*in vitro*). Levels of PEA are not known to influence neuron response to serotonin, GABA or glutamate. Trace amines may activate sigma receptors (*in vitro*), which modulate potassium and calcium channels. Altering the level of ions inside of neurons may change their action potential and firing rate.

Receptors:

The trace amine-associated receptors (TAARs) are a recently discovered class of receptors that respond to various trace amines. Most TAARs activity is the result of second messenger signaling through cyclic adenosine monophosphate (cAMP) and protein phosphorylation. TAARs are found in the CNS and in the periphery are primarily found in the gastrointestinal tract, lung, and kidneys. In other mammals, some TAARs may serve as olfactory chemoreceptors and may respond to stimulation by odorous amines. Research continues into the function of TAARs and their ligands as not all TAAR subtypes respond to known trace amines. Mutations or single nucleotide polymorphisms in the nine genes coding for TAARs may affect receptor conformation or function, which may increase susceptibility risk for schizophrenia or bipolar disorders. In vitro and in vivo studies indicate:

- TAAR1

  - Intracellular expression
  - Binds to tyramine and PEA with greatest affinity; also binds other trace amines, catecholamines and serotonin
  - May modulate catecholamines and serotonin by altering cell membrane transport or receptor function
    - In vitro studies indicate that PEA binding to TAAR1 inhibits reuptake and induces release of dopamine, norepinephrine and serotonin from neurons
  - Expressed in the CNS and in leukocytes, gastrointestinal tract, lung, and kidneys
    - has been shown in vitro to assist leukocyte chemotaxis towards trace amines; binding of trace amines to TAAR1 in leukocytes has been shown in vitro to promote cytokine release
  - Binds with amphetamines and psychotropic agents (ergot alkaloids, bromocriptine, lisuride, D-lysergic acid diethylamide (LSD), 3,4-methylenedioxy-methamphetamine [MDMA or ecstasy])
  - Interacts with the thyroid hormone derivative 3-iodothyronamines, which may affect temperature regulation and cardiac contractility (*in vivo*)

- TAAR2

  - Binds to trace amines
  - Has been shown in vitro to assist leukocyte chemotaxis towards trace amines; binding of trace amines to TAAR2 in leukocytes has been shown in vitro to promote cytokine release
  - Nonsense mutation may contribute to some cases of schizophrenia

- TAAR5

  - Function in humans unknown

- TAAR6

  - Expressed in the amygdala of the brain and in leukocytes, kidneys
  - SNP has been associated with increased familial susceptibility to schizophrenia in those of European or African-American ancestry

- TAAR8

  - Expressed in the amygdala of the brain and in leukocytes, kidneys

- TAAR9

  - Expressed in pituitary and in leukocytes, kidney and skeletal muscle

Consider:

- Phenylalanine precursor status (**Plasma** or **Urine Amino Acids**)

- Selenium status (**RBC Elements**)

- Glutathione status (**Glutathione; erythrocytes**)

- Oxidative stress (**DNA Oxidative Damage Assay/8-OHdG**)

References:

Berry, M D (2007)
The potential of trace amines and their receptors for treating neurological and psychiatric diseases.
Reviews on recent clinical trials vol. 2 (1) p. 3-19

Berry, Mark D (2004)
Mammalian central nervous system trace amines. Pharmacologic amphetamines, physiologic neuromodulators.
Journal of neurochemistry vol. 90 (2) p. 257-71

Husebye, E S; Boe, A S; Rorsman, F; Kämpe, O; Aakvaag, A et al. (2000)
Inhibition of aromatic L-amino acid decarboxylase activity by human autoantibodies.
Clinical and experimental immunology vol. 120 (3) p. 420-3

Kusaga, Akira (2002)
Decreased beta-phenylethylamine in urine of children with attention deficit hyperactivity disorder and autistic disorder.
No to hattatsu. Brain and development vol. 34 (3) p. 243-8

Ledonne, Ada; Berretta, Nicola; Davoli, Alessandro; Rizzo, Giada Ricciardo; Bernardi, Giorgio et al. (2011)
Electrophysiological effects of trace amines on mesencephalic dopaminergic neurons.
Frontiers in systems neuroscience vol. 5 p. 56

Licata, Angelo A.; Radfar, Nezam; Bartter, Frederic C.; Bou, Ernestina (1978)
The urinary excretion of phosphoethanolamine in diseases other than hypophosphatasia
The American Journal of Medicine vol. 64 (1) p. 133-138

Narang, Deepak et al. (2011)
Trace Amines and Their Relevance to Psychiatry and Neurology: A Brief Overview
Bulletin of Clinical Psychopharmacology 2011;21:73-79

Tang, Ya-Li; Wang, Shih-Wei; Lin, Shyh-Mirn (2008)
Both inorganic and organic selenium supplements can decrease brain monoamine oxidase B enzyme activity in adult rats.
The British journal of nutrition vol. 100 (3) p. 660-5

Xie, Zhihua; Miller, Gregory M. (2008)
-Phenylethylamine Alters Monoamine Transporter Function via Trace Amine-Associated Receptor 1: Implication for Modulatory Roles of Trace Amines in Brain
J. Pharmacol. Exp. Ther. vol. 325 (2) p. 617-628

Zucchi, R; Chiellini, G; Scanlan, T S; Grandy, D K (2006)
Trace amine-associated receptors and their ligands.
British journal of pharmacology vol. 149 (8) p. 967-78

Taurine (2-aminoethane-sulfonic acid)

The essential amino acid taurine is most abundant in the brain, spinal cord, leukocytes, heart, muscle cells, and retina. Taurine promotes neural development in both the embryonic and adult brain. Taurine acts as a neuromodulator and exerts, *in vitro*, an inhibitory effect on the firing rate of central nervous system (CNS) neurons. Taurine has been shown in human and animal studies to have mild anti-convulsant effects.

In the CNS taurine regulates the levels of electrolytes within neurons; the level of ions such as calcium, magnesium and potassium within neurons alters the action potential (firing rate) in the nerve cell. Taurine's effects in the CNS may vary by taurine concentration, brain region and neurotransmitter receptor type. Taurine has antioxidant properties; it stabilizes the electron transport chain within the mitochondria and inhibits the generation of reactive oxygen species. Oxidative stress (the production of radical oxygen species) is associated with many neurologic disorders. Taurine does not cross the blood brain barrier (BBB) easily and must be synthesized within the CNS.

Effects:

Decreased taurine levels may occur due to dietary insufficiency or digestion and absorption issues in the gastrointestinal tract. Decreased CNS taurine synthesis has been reported in individuals with autoimmune and neurodegenerative diseases, including rheumatoid arthritis, Parkinson's disease, Alzheimer's disease, and motor neuron diseases such as amyotrophic lateral sclerosis (ALS). Low levels of taurine during development may result in abnormal brain development. A low urinary taurine due

to a renal clearance disorder may occasionally mask an elevated plasma taurine level.

Excess urinary taurine levels may result from inherited renal defects, liver disease, heart disease or radiation injury. High plasma taurine may be associated with stress reactions, depression and psychosis. Plasma and urinary taurine may increase due to liver inflammation or disease. Oral supplementation may raise taurine levels. Taurine is an ingredient in many "energy drinks" and taurine supplements may be used by athletes. Taurine supplements may be used to treat seizure disorders, autism and attention deficit-hyperactivity disorder (ADHD). Patients with Cushing's disease may have elevated urinary taurine levels, but low plasma levels. Patients with autism may have elevated urine taurine, glycine and alanine with low glutamate.

Synthesis and Metabolism:

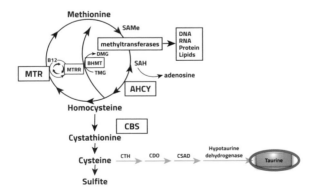

Taurine synthesis from cysteine.
The methylation pathway (as it is commonly known) synthesizes cysteine behind the blood-brain barrier, and is a precursor for the antioxidants taurine and glutathione.

Legend: AHCY = adenosylhomocysteinase; BHMT = betaine-homocysteine methyltransferase; CBS; CTH = Cystathionine gamma-lyase; CDO = Cysteine dioxygenase; CSAD = cysteine sulfinate decarboxylase; MTR = methionine synthase; MTRR = methionine synthase reductase; MTHFR = methylenetetrahydrofolate reductase; SUOX

Taurine may be obtained from the diet, however taurine does not easily pass the BBB. Taurine synthesis occurs mainly in the liver and the CNS. Adequate taurine synthesis in the brain requires normal activity of what is now commonly referred to as the methylation pathway, as methionine must be metabolized to synthesize cysteine behind the BBB. Taurine may then be synthesized from cysteine.

In the first step of taurine synthesis, cysteine dioxygenase (CDO) oxidizes cysteine to cysteine sulfinate. Cysteine sulfinate has two possible metabolic fates. It may be transaminated by aspartate aminotransferase (AAT) to pyruvate and sulfate, or it may be decarboxylated by cysteine sulfinate decarboxylase (CSAD) to hypotaurine. Humans in general have low CSAD activity. Both CDO and CSAD require a pyridoxal phosphate (vitamin B6) cofactor. Rate-limiting factors for enzymatic conversion include age and gender (male enzymes are more active than female). High protein diets increase CDO but decrease CSAD activity in animal studies. This response to a high protein diet favors sulfate formation, but not taurine synthesis.

In the final synthetic step, hypotaurine is converted to taurine by hypotaurine dehydrogenase, which requires a molybdenum cofactor (heme, a cofactor for rat hypotaurine dehydrogenase, has not been confirmed in humans). Cysteamine, the product of coenzyme A metabolism, may also be converted into hypotaurine by cysteamine dioxygenase (2-aminoethanethiol dioxygenase [ADO]), which requires an iron cofactor. *In vitro* studies indicate that the conversion of hypotaurine into taurine may be the rate-limiting step of taurine synthesis in astroglia and neurons. *In vi-*

tro studies also indicate that taurine synthesis is stimulated in neurons by hypertonic media conditions (high electrolyte levels). Hypo-osmotic media increased taurine release from cultured brain cells. Osmotic changes in the CNS are known to occur due to ischemia, trauma, hypoglycemia, hypoxia, hepatic encephalopathy or hyponatremia.

Taurine is actively transported into cells by a specific sodium-dependant transporter (TauT). Genetic defects in TauT have been associated with decreased tissue taurine levels, blindness, decreased fertility and poor exercise capacity. Transporter activity may also be affected by electrolyte concentrations, action potentials, and second-messenger cellular signals.

Taurine has been shown to increase the expression of glutamic acid decarboxylase (GAD), which synthesizes GABA from glutamate (*in vitro* and *in vivo* animal studies). Taurine is a potent regulator of intracellular calcium homeostasis. Endogenous taurine in retina and nerve cells inhibits glutamate-induced calcium influx and may protect against glutamate exitotoxicity. Through the modulation of calcium channel influx, taurine inhibits the release of cytochrome C from mitochondria, which prevents cell apoptosis. Taurine, when injected daily, improved learning and normalized acetylcholine metabolism in manganese-exposed rats. Taurine administration in rodents has been shown to have anxiety-reducing and anti-depressive effects in animal studies, these effects may be dose dependent.

Taurine is excreted via urine and bile; the kidney regulates plasma levels by altering rates of renal tubular reabsorption. The amount of taurine excreted daily is affected by various factors including genetics, age, gender, diet, renal function and medical conditions.

Receptors:

No specific neuro-active taurine receptor has yet been identified, but taurine has been shown in vitro and in vivo, to affect other neurotransmitter receptors. Taurine may potentiate N-methyl-D-aspartate (NMDA), gamma-aminobutyrate A (GABA-A) and glycine receptors. Taurine may compete with glycine for glycine receptor sites.

Taurine may influence presynaptic N-methyl-D-aspartate (NMDA) receptor signaling, and is known to bind with gamma-aminobutyric acid (GABA)-A/B receptors (in vitro and in vivo animal studies). Glycine must also bind to NMDA receptors to activate them and taurine may compete with glycine for NMDAR access. Strong taurine activation of a group of GABA-A receptors in the rodent thalamus has been recently documented. The thalamus is involved in "behavioral state control" and regulates transitions between sleep and wakefulness.

The effects of taurine on various receptors may vary by taurine concentration, brain region and neurotransmitter receptor type.

Consider:

- Renal function (**Creatinine Clearance Test**)

- Serum electrolyte status (**Serum Elements**)

- Intracellular electrolyte status (**RBC Elements**)

- Methionine metabolism and methylation pathways (**Plasma Methylation Profile, DNA Methylation Pathway**)

- Oxidative stress/8OH-dG (**DNA Oxidative Damage Assay**)

References:

Cornell Chronicle (2014)
Scientists close in on taurine's activity in the brain (Red Bull drinkers, take note)
Cornell Chronicle • 312 College Ave., Ithaca, NY 14850
http://news.cornell.edu/stories/2008/02/scientists-close-taurines-activity-brain retrieved 10 September 2014

Faggiano, Antongiulio; Melis, Daniela; Alfieri, Raffaele; De Martino, MariaCristina; Filippella, Mariagiovanna et al. (2005)
Sulfur amino acids in Cushing's disease: insight in homocysteine and taurine levels in patients with active and cured disease.
The Journal of clinical endocrinology and metabolism vol. 90 (12) p. 6616-22

Han, X; Patters, A B; Jones, D P; Zelikovic, I; Chesney, R W
The taurine transporter: mechanisms of regulation.
Acta physiologica (Oxford, England) vol. 187 (1-2) p. 61-73

Ivan K S Yap; Manya Angley (2010)
Urinary metabolic phenotyping differentiates children with autism from their unaffected siblings and age-matched controls.
Journal of proteome research vol. 9 (6) p. 2996 - 3004

Jerkins, Ann A.; Jones, Deborah D.; Kohlhepp, Edwin A. (1998)
Cysteine Sulfinic Acid Decarboxylase mRNA Abundance Decreases in Rats Fed a High-Protein Diet
J. Nutr. vol. 128 (11) p. 1890-1895

Lourenco and Camilo (2002)

Taurine: a conditionally essential amino acid in humans? An overview in health and disease.
Nutr. Hosp. (2002) XVII (6) 262-270
ISSN 0212-1611 • CODEN NUHOEQ S.V.R. 318

Lu, Cai-Ling; Tang, Shen; Meng, Zhi-Juan; He, Yi-Yuan; Song, Ling-Yong et al. (2014)
Taurine improves the spatial learning and memory ability impaired by sub-chronic manganese exposure.
Journal of biomedical science vol. 21 p. 51

Menzie, Janet; Pan, Chunliu; Prentice, Howard; Wu, Jang-Yen (2014)
Taurine and central nervous system disorders.
Amino acids vol. 46 (1) p. 31-46

Ripps, Harris; Shen, Wen (2012)
Review: taurine: a "very essential" amino acid.
Molecular vision vol. 18 p. 2673-86

Stipanuk, M H; Ueki, I; Dominy, J E; Simmons, C R; Hirschberger, L L (2009)
Cysteine dioxygenase: a robust system for regulation of cellular cysteine levels.
Amino acids vol. 37 (1) p. 55-63

Ueki, Iori; Stipanuk, Martha H. (2007)
Enzymes of the Taurine Biosynthetic Pathway Are Expressed in Rat Mammary Gland
J. Nutr. vol. 137 (8) p. 1887-1894

Taurine biosynthesis by neurons and astrocytes.
Vitvitsky, Victor; Garg, Sanjay K; Banerjee, Ruma (2011)
The Journal of biological chemistry vol. 286 (37) p. 32002-10

Glycine

Glycine is a non-essential dietary amino acid. Glycine signaling contributes to a variety of motor and sensory functions, primarily pain perception.

Glycine has an inhibitory effect when binding to glycine receptors in the spinal cord, brainstem or retina, and is considered inhibitory in the CNS, though glycine synapses may be excitatory in the immature brain (animal studies). In the brain, glycine is an essential cofactor with glutamate for N-methyl-D-aspartate (NDMA) receptor excitatory signaling. The release of glycine by glial cells and the presence of glycine transporters on those cells suggest that glycine may also act as a neuromodulator.

Effects:

Decreased urinary glycine may occur due to impaired renal clearance or toxicant exposure. Glycine is required for glutathione synthesis and purine synthesis for DNA or RNA. Glycine does not cross the blood brain barrier easily. Endogenous and xenobiotic organic acids and aromatic acids are conjugated to glycine for excretion in the urine. In the CNS, glycine conjugation occurs in the mitochondria and provides a mechanism to remove aromatic acid toxicants such as benzoic acid. Glycine supplements have been used to improve sleep quality and used in conjunction with pharmaceutical supports for schizophrenia.

Excess glycine is metabolized by the mitochondria using the enzyme glycine decarboxylase into 5,10,-methylene tetrahydrofolate, CO-2 and ammonia. Glycine decarbooxylase is commonly called the glycine cleavage complex (GCC); it is comprised of four different proteins and requires pyridoxal phosphate (B-6) and tetrahydrofolate cofactors. Genetic defects in the GCC may result in glycine encephalopathy. This condition is characterized by nonketotic hyperglycinemia (NKH) and elevated urinary glycine. Animal studies indicate that elevated glycine levels may severely impair energy synthesis and use in the CNS. The elevated levels of glycine in the CNS result in intellectual disability, poor muscle tone, chorea (involuntary movements), respiratory or feeding difficulties. Most cases are diagnosed during infancy. Occasionally a patient will have a milder, atypical form of disease, with onset from late infancy into adulthood. Glycine supplements may be used in conjunction with pharmaceutical supports for schizophrenia or psychosis, and may result in elevated urinary glycine. Combinations of glycine with antipsychotics or glycine transport inhibitors have improved symptoms in some schizophrenia patients, and increased glycine serum levels have been reported in schizophrenia patients responsive to antipsychotics.

Synthesis and Metabolism:

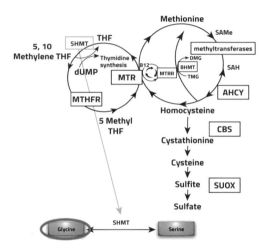

Glycine is synthesized in the cell cytoplasm via serine hydroxymethyltransferase (cSHMT) using a pyridoxal phosphate (B6) cofactor. In the liver, glycine may be synthesized using glycine synthase and NADH. There is no specific transporter across the blood-brain barrier (BBB) for glycine, but there are glycine-specific transporters that take glycine into cells and remove it from neural synapses. There are two types of glycine transporters, GLYT-1 and GLYT-2. Mapping studies indicate that GLYT-1 is primarily associated with astroglia cells, and is found in the same CNS regions as glycine receptors. GLYT-2 is primarily associated with neurons. The glycine transporters act as regulators of glycine, which has dual functions: it acts as:

- an inhibitory neurotransmitter at glycinergic synapses and in the spinal cord

- as a modulator of neuron excitation, mediated by NMDA receptors at glutamate neuron synapses

The two major subtypes of glycine transporters, GlyT1 and GlyT2, have been linked to the pathogenesis and/or treatment of central and peripheral nervous system disorders, including schizophrenia and related affective and cognitive disturbances, alcohol dependence, pain, epilepsy, breathing disorders and startle disease (also known as hyperekplexia). Sarcosine may act as a GlyT1 inhibitor. Animal studies indicate that GlyT2 may play an important role in clearing glycine from the spinal cord, and may play further roles both in bladder hyperactivity and in the perception of pain.

Receptors:

Glycine receptors are known primarily through their function in spinal circuits; they are important in both motor control and pain perception. Glycine receptors are also found in various areas of the brain. Genetic variations in the glycine receptor may contribute to seizure disorders, and genetic variation in the NDMA receptor may affect neuron excitability and plasticity. Genetic disorders of glycine, gamma-aminobutyric acid (GABA), and serine metabolism are associated with seizure disorders, as are genetic defects in GABA and glycine receptor function. Mutations of glycine receptor subunits have been associated with hereditary hyperekplexia (startle disease) and some types of autism. Studies with knockout mice indicate that mutations in glycine receptors may affect the function of the hippocampus and, in addition to causing seizures, may alter memory and cognition. The three primary endogenous agonists for glycine receptors are, in order of receptor affinity: glycine, β-alanine and taurine. Caffeine has been shown to inhibit glycine receptors in vitro.

Consider:

- Serine levels (**Amino Acids**)

- Transsulfuration pathway integrity and methylation capacity (**Plasma Methylation Profile**)

- Glutathione status (**Glutathione; erythrocytes**)

References:

Avila, Ariel; Nguyen, Laurent; Rigo, Jean-Michel (2013)
Glycine receptors and brain development.
Frontiers in cellular neuroscience vol. 7 p. 184

Badenhorst CP; Erasmus E; van der Sluis R; Nortje C; van Dijk AA (2014)
A new perspective on the importance of glycine conjugation in the metabolism of aromatic acids.
Drug Metab Rev. 2014; 46(3):343-61

Betz, H; Gomeza, J; Armsen, W; Scholze, P; Eulenburg, V (2006)
Glycine transporters: essential regulators of synaptic transmission.
Biochemical Society transactions vol. 34 (Pt 1) p. 55-8

Busanello, Estela Natacha Brandt; Moura, Alana Pimentel; Viegas, Carolina Maso; Zanatta, Ângela; da Costa Ferreira, Gustavo et al. (2010)
Neurochemical evidence that glycine induces bioenergetical dysfunction
Neurochemistry International vol. 56 (8) p. 948-954

Duan, Lei; Yang, Jaeyoung; Slaughter, Malcolm M (2009)
Caffeine inhibition of ionotropic glycine receptors.
The Journal of physiology vol. 587 (Pt 16) p. 4063-75

Glycine receptors. (2009).
British Journal of Pharmacology,158 (Suppl 1), S117–S118. doi:10.1111/j.1476-5381.2009.00502_6.x

Harvey, Robert J.; Yee, Benjamin K. (2013)

Glycine transporters as novel therapeutic targets in schizophrenia, alcohol dependence and pain
Nature Publishing Group, a division of Macmillan Publishers Limited. All Rights Reserved. vol. 12 (11) p. 866-885

Legendre, P. (2001)
The glycinergic inhibitory synapse
Cellular and Molecular Life Sciences vol. 58 (5) p. 760-793

Paul, Steven M. (2002)
GABA and Glycine
Neuropsychopharmacology: The Fifth Generation of Progress Editors:
Lippincott, Williams, & Wilkins, Philadelphia, Pennsylvania, 2002

Satoru Yoshikawa, Tomohiko Oguchi (2012)
Glycine transporter type 2 (GlyT2) inhibitor ameliorates bladder overactivity and nociceptive behavior in rats.
European urology vol. 62 (4) p. 704 - 12

Winkelmann, Aline; Maggio, Nicola; Eller, Joanna; Caliskan, Gürsel; Semtner, Marcus et al. (2014)
Changes in neural network homeostasis trigger neuropsychiatric symptoms.
The Journal of clinical investigation vol. 124 (2) p. 696-711

Yang, Charles R.; Svensson, Kjell A. (2008)
Allosteric modulation of NMDA receptor via elevation of brain glycine and d-serine: The therapeutic potentials for schizophrenia.
Pharmacology & Therapeutics vol. 120 (3) p. 317-332

Histamine

Histamine is derived from the essential amino acid histidine. Histamine mediates numerous biologic reactions by binding with its receptors in the brain and in the body. Histamine is one of the most important neurotransmitters to stimulate and maintain arousal in the central nervous system (CNS). Histamine-acetylcholine signaling interactions contribute to wakefulness (arousal), attention, circadian rhythms, appetite control, learning, memory and emotion. Histamine may also bind to N-methyl-D-aspartate (NMDA) receptors. Histamine may affect the secretion of posterior and anterior pituitary hormones, including the release of prolactin. Histamine may also contribute to the stress-related release of adrenocorticotropic hormone (ACTH).

In the peripheral nervous system, histamine signaling affects smooth muscle tone, digestion, gut motility and immune responses. Histamine is a mediator of allergic Type I hypersensitivity reactions. Histamine released during allergic reactions may result in itching, flushing, hives, vomiting, syncope (fainting), anaphylaxis or shock.

Effects:

Decreased histamine levels in the CNS may result from nicotinic acetylcholine receptor and serotonin signaling. Sedatives such as ethanol, tetrahydrocannabinol (THC), barbiturates and benzodiazepines may also decrease histamine levels. Low levels of CNS histamine may also contribute to Tourette's syndrome, narcolepsy and other hypersomnia (sleep) disorders. Alterations in CNS histamine levels may contribute to age-related neurodegenerative diseases such as Parkinson's disease and Alzheimer's disease. Current research indicates that increases or decreases in CNS histamine levels may occur locally in specific brain areas during neurodegenerative diseases.

Low levels of the precursor essential amino acid histidine may occur from poor diet or digestive disorders. Two rare genetic disorders, histidine ammonia-lyase deficiency or histidine decarboxylase deficiency, may prevent the conversion of histidine to histamine. These enzymatic defects may elevate histidine levels and may result in lower histamine levels. Pyridoxal phosphate (Vitamin B-6) deficiency may inhibit histidine decarboxylase function.

Excess histamine may result from medications. Animal studies indicate that morphine, clozapine, olanzapine, methylphenidate, atomoxetine and other pharmaceuticals may increase histamine release in the CNS. Increased populations of CNS mast cells and histamine levels have been associated with multiple sclerosis (MS). Increased levels of histamine metabolites have been found in the cerebrospinal fluid of schizophrenic patients. Increased histamine synthesis has been associated with stim-

ulation of dopamine, opioid and NMDA receptors. Alterations in CNS histamine levels may contribute to age-related neurodegenerative diseases such as Parkinson's disease and Alzheimer's disease. Current research indicates that increases or decreases in CNS histamine levels may occur locally in specific brain areas during neurodegenerative diseases.

Patients with allergies or mastocytosis may have higher plasma histamine levels. Certain bacteria in the gastrointestinal microbiome may synthesize histamine, and some patients with gastric carcinoid tumors may have elevated histamine levels. Elevated plasma histamine and diamine oxidase (DAO) deficiency have been associated with inflammatory bowel disease (IBD), allergic enteropathy, colorectal cancers, and food allergy. DAO is a copper-binding enzyme.

Synthesis and Metabolism:

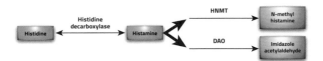

Histamine is synthesized by immune cells, platelets, histamine neurons, and gastrointestinal enterochromaffin cells. Histidine is converted into histamine by histidine decarboxylase, which requires a pyridoxal phosphate (vitamin B6) cofactor. Deficient function of histamine decarboxylase has been associated with symptoms of Tourette's syndrome. Histamine is stored in neuron vesicles until released. Histamine synthesis may be influenced by oxidative stress, glucocorticoids, gastrin and other neuroactive peptides. Histamine is inactivated in the synapse by extracellular histamine N-methyltransferase (HNMT).

HNMT requires S-adenosyl methionine (SAM) as a methyl donor. Diamine oxidase (DAO) degrades histamine, and one of its metabolite is neuro-active. Monoamine oxidase B (MAO-B) may further degrade histamine metabolites.

Approximately one percent of the population has histamine intolerance, caused by reduced diamine oxidase (DAO) activity. DAO degrades ingested histamine, and may scavenge extracellular histamine in the body. Symptoms of DAO deficiency may resemble allergic hypersensitivity reactions, but are caused by the ingestion of histamine-rich foods, alcohol or pharmaceuticals that release histamine. Symptoms may include diffuse epigastric discomfort, colic, flatulence, diarrhea, nasal congestion, asthma-like wheezing, hypotension, arrhythmia, urticaria (hives), pruritus (itching), flushing, headaches (migraine or cluster). Deficiencies of DAO or aldehyde dehydrogenase may also decrease levels of the neuroactive metabolite of histamine, imidazoleacetic acid-ribotide (IAA-RP). In the CNS, histamine neurons are located in the posterior hypothalamus, and project their fibers to most regions of the brain. Histamine neurons also metabolize a variety of other neurotransmitters in addition to histamine.

Receptors:

Histamine binds with different groups of histamine receptors and may also bind to N-methyl-D-aspartate (NMDA) receptors.

- H_1

  - Widespread distribution in the brain; mediates excitatory responses; may contribute to wakefulness and cognition
  - Expressed in smooth muscle and endothelial cells
  - Contributes to IgE Type I hypersensitivity reactions

- H_2

  - Expressed in areas of the brain; may modulate action potential of neurons
  - Expressed on white blood cells
  - Stimulation of H2 receptors on parietal cells induces the release of hydrochloric acid in the stomach

- H_3

  - Exclusively expressed in neurons and modulate neurotransmission; inhibitory; regulate the release of monoamines, acetylcholine and histamine
  - Expressed in pre-synaptic and post-synaptic neurons in different parts of the brain
  - Found in proximity to dopamine receptors in the basal ganglia of the brain

- H_4

  - Expressed on mast cells, eosinophils, T-cells, and dendritic cells
  - Regulate immunity

Consider:

- Copper status (**RBC Elements**)

- Histidine precursor status (**Plasma Amino Acids**)

- Oxidative stress (**DNA Oxidative Damage Assay/8-OHdG**)

- Methylation pathway activity (**Plasma Methylation Profile, DNA Methylation Pathway**)

References:

Blandina, Patrizio; Efoudebe, Marcel; Cenni, Gabriele; Mannaioni, Pierfrancesco; Passani, Maria Beatrice (2004)
Acetylcholine, Histamine, and Cognition: Two Sides of the Same Coin
Learn. Mem. vol. 11 (1) p. 1-8

Bowen, R.(2008)
Histamine and Histamine receptors.
Colorado State University
http://www.vivo.colostate.edu/hbooks/path-phys/endocrine/otherendo/histamine.html
Accessed 15 January 2015

Castellan Baldan, Lissandra; Williams, Kyle A; Gallezot, Jean-Dominique; Pogorelov, Vladimir; Rapanelli, Maximiliano et al. (2014) Histidine decarboxylase deficiency causes tourette syndrome: parallel findings in humans and mice. *Neuron vol.* 81 (1) p. 77-90

Devaraj, Sridevi; Hemarajata, Peera; Versalovic, James (2013) The Human Gut Microbiome and Body Metabolism: Implications for Obesity and Diabetes *Clin. Chem.* vol. 59 (4) p. 617-628

Fell, Matthew J; Katner, Jason S; Rasmussen, Kurt; Nikolayev, Alexander; Kuo, Ming-Shang et al. (2012) Typical and atypical antipsychotic drugs increase extracellular histamine levels in the rat medial prefrontal cortex: contribution of histamine h(1) receptor blockade. *Frontiers in psychiatry* vol. 3 p. 49

Friedman, B S; Steinberg, S C; Meggs, W J; Kaliner, M A; Frieri, M et al. (1989) Analysis of plasma histamine levels in patients with mast cell disorders. *The American journal of medicine* vol. 87 (6) p. 649-54

Hofstra, Claudia L.; Desai, Pragnya J.; Thurmond, Robin L.; Fung-Leung, Wai-Ping (2003) Histamine H4 Receptor Mediates Chemotaxis and Calcium Mobilization of Mast Cells *J. Pharmacol. Exp. Ther.* vol. 305 (3) p. 1212-1221

Horner, Weldon E.; Johnson, David E.; Schmidt, Anne W.; Rollema, Hans (2007) Methylphenidate and atomoxetine increase histamine release in rat prefrontal cortex *European Journal of Pharmacology* vol. 558 (1) p. 96-97

KAROVI OVA, J. and KOHAJDOVA, Z. Biogenic Amines in Food

Chem. Pap. 59(1)70—79 (2005)

Kimura, K; Adachi, M; Kubo, K; Ikemoto, Y (1999) The basal plasma histamine level and eosinophil count in allergic and non-allergic patients. *Fukuoka igaku zasshi = Hukuoka acta medica* vol. 90 (12) p. 457-63

Maintz, Laura; Novak, Natalija (2007) Histamine and histamine intolerance *Am J Clin Nutr* vol. 85 (5) p. 1185-1196

Oishi, R; Nishibori, M; Itoh, Y; Saeki, K (1986) Diazepam-induced decrease in histamine turnover in mouse brain. *European journal of pharmacology* vol. 124 (3) p. 337-42

Prell, George D; Martinelli, Giorgio P; Holstein, Gay R; Matuli -Adami , Jasenka; Watanabe, Kyoichi A et al. (2004) Imidazoleacetic acid-ribotide: an endogenous ligand that stimulates imidazol(in)e receptors. *Proceedings of the National Academy of Sciences of the United States of America* vol. 101 (37) p. 13677-82

Scammell, Thomas E; Mochizuki, Takatoshi (2009) Is low histamine a fundamental cause of sleepiness in narcolepsy and idiopathic hypersomnia? *Sleep vol.* 32 (2) p. 133-4

Schwartz, Jean-Charles; Arrang, Jean-Michael; Garbarg, Monique. (2002) Histamine Neuropsychopharmacology – 5th Generation of Progress Lippincott, Williams, & Wilkins, Philadelphia, Pennsylvania, 2002

Molecular and cellular analysis of human histamine receptor subtypes. Seifert, Roland; Strasser, Andrea; Schneider, Erich H; Neumann, Detlef; Dove, Stefan et al. (2013)

Trends in pharmacological sciences vol. 34 (1) p. 33-58

Shan, Ling; Swaab, Dick F.; Bao, Ai-Min. (2013)
Neuronal histaminergic system in aging and age-related neurodegenerative disorders
Experimental Gerontology. Volume 48, Issue 7, July 2013, Pages 603–607

Yanai, Kazuhiko; Tashiro, Manabu (2007)
The physiological and pathophysiological roles of neuronal histamine: an insight from human positron emission tomography studies.
Pharmacology & therapeutics vol. 113 (1) p. 1-15

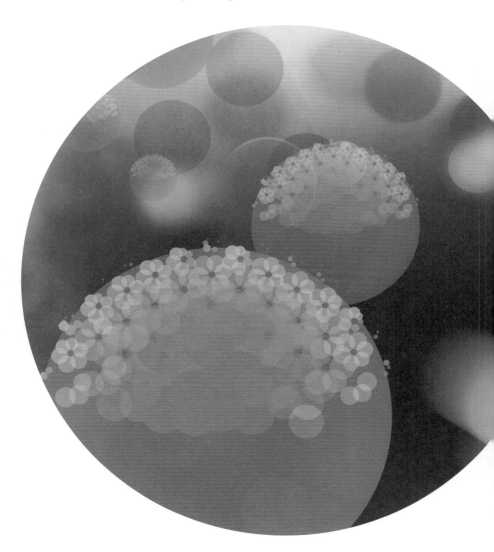

Document References:

....

Agency for Toxic Substances and Disease Registry (ATSDR). 2004. Toxicological profile for cesium. Atlanta, GA: U.S. Department of Health and Human Services, Public Health Service.

Agency for Toxic Substances and Disease Registry (ATSDR) Public Health Statements.
Toxic Substances Portal
http://www.atsdr.cdc.gov/substances/ ToxChemicalClasses.asp
Accessed February 2015

American Association for Clinical Chemistry
www.labtestsonline.org
Accessed November/December 2014

Aoki, Y (2001)
Polychlorinated biphenyls, polychlorinated dibenzo-p-dioxins, and polychlorinated dibenzofurans as endocrine disrupt-ers--what we have learned from Yusho disease.
Environmental research vol. 86 (1) p. 2-11

Asano, Yasunari; Hiramoto, Tetsuya; Nishino, Ryo; Aiba, Yuji; Kimura, Tae et al. (2012)
Critical role of gut microbiota in the produc-tion of biologically active, free catechol-amines in the gut lumen of mice
Am J Physiol Gastrointest Liver Physiol vol. 303 (11) p. G1288-1295

Barber, D.S.; Hancock, S.K.; McNally, A.M.; Hinckley, J.; Binder, E. et al. (2007)
Neurological effects of acute uranium expo-sure with and without stress
NeuroToxicology vol. 28 (6) p. 1110-1119

Bauer, M; Heinz, A; Whybrow, P.C.

Thyroid hormones, serotonin and mood: of synergy and significance in the adult brain
(2002)
Nature Publishing Group vol. 7 (2)

Becker, Danielle A; Balcer, Laura J; Galetta, Steven L (2012)
The Neurological Complications of Nutritional Deficiency following Bariatric Surgery.
Journal of obesity vol. 2012 p. 608534

Benton, David (2002)
Selenium intake, mood and other aspects of psychological functioning.
Nutritional neuroscience vol. 5 (6) p. 363-74

Bienenstock, J. (2012).
Commensal communication to the brain: pathways and behavioral consequences.
Microbial ecology in health and disease, 23. doi:10.3402/mehd.v23i0.19007

Blakemore, Colin and Jennett, Shelia
The Oxford Companion To The Body
(2001)
Copyright 2012 Practitioner Medical Publishing.

Blum, Ian D; Zhu, Lei; Moquin, Luc; Kokoeva, Maia V; Gratton, Alain et al. (2015)
A highly tunable dopaminergic oscillator generates ultradian rhythms of behavioral arousal
eLife vol. 3 p. e05105

Borges Fernandes, Luciana Cristina; Campos Câmara, Carlos; Soto-Blanco, Benito (2012)

Anticonvulsant Activity of Extracts of Plectranthus barbatus Leaves in Mice. *Evidence-based complementary and alternative medicine* : eCAM vol. 2012 p. 860153

Bottiglieri, Teodoro (2002) S-Adenosyl-L-methionine (SAMe): from the bench to the bedside--molecular basis of a pleiotrophic molecule *Am J Clin Nutr* vol. 76 (5) p. 1151S-1157

Braniste, Viorica; Al-Asmakh, Maha; Kowal, Czeslawa; Anuar, Farhana; Abbaspour, Afrouz et al. (2014) The gut microbiota influences blood-brain barrier permeability in mice. *Science translational medicine* vol. 6 (263) p. 263ra158

Bradley, Paul M.; Barber, Larry B.; Duris, Joseph W.; Foreman, William T.; Furlong, Edward T. et al. (2014) Riverbank filtration potential of pharmaceuticals in a wastewater-impacted stream *Environmental Pollution* vol. 193 p. 173-180

Bresden, Dale E. (2014) Reversal of cognitive decline: A novel therapeutic program. *AGING*, Vol 6, No 9 , pp 707-717 Accessed 25 February 2015

Brinton, Roberta Diaz; Thompson, Richard F; Foy, Michael R; Baudry, Michel; Wang, Junming et al. (2008) Progesterone receptors: form and function in brain. *Frontiers in neuroendocrinology* vol. 29 (2) p. 313-39

Byrne, John H., Editor Neuroscience Online an electronic textbook for the neurosciences. Accessed 10 December 2014

Centers for Disease Control and Prevention Emergency Preparedness and Response Chemical Emergencies *http://www.bt.cdc.gov/chemical/index.asp* Accessed February 2015

Centers for Disease Control

Environmental Health Hazards & Health Effects Harmful Algal Blooms (HABs) *http://www.cdc.gov/nceh/ciguatera/* Accessed 10 February 2015

Choi, Anna l.; Sun, Guifan; Zhang, Ying; Grandjean, Philippe. Developmental Fluoride Neurotoxicity: A Systematic Review and Meta-Analysis *Environ Health Perspect*; DOI:10.1289/ ehp.1104912

Costes, Léa M M; Boeckxstaens, Guy E; de Jonge, Wouter J; Cailotto, Cathy (2013) Neural networks in intestinal immunoregulation. *Organogenesis* vol. 9 (3) p. 216-23 July 1, 2013.

Coughtrie, Michael W. H.; Johnston, Laura E. (2001) Interactions between Dietary Chemicals and Human Sulfotransferases - Molecular Mechanisms and Clinical Significance *Drug Metab. Dispos.* vol. 29 (4) p. 522-528

Davison, Karen M; Kaplan, Bonnie J (2013) Nutrient- and non-nutrient-based natural health product (NHP) use in adults with mood disorders: prevalence, characteristics and potential for exposure to adverse events. *BMC complementary and alternative medicine* vol. 13 p. 80

Davison, Karen M; Kaplan, Bonnie J (2012) Nutrient Intakes Are Correlated With Overall Psychiatric Functioning in Adults With Mood Disorders. Can J Psychiatry. 2012;57(2):85–92

de la Monte, Suzanne M; Tong, Ming (2009) Mechanisms of nitrosamine-mediated neurodegeneration: potential relevance to sporadic Alzheimer's disease. *Journal of Alzheimer's disease : JAD* vol. 17 (4) p. 817-25

Desai, Vishal; Kaler, Stephen G (2008) Role of copper in human neurological disorders

Am J Clin Nutr vol. 88 (3) p. 855S-858

Dinan, T. G., & Cryan, J. F. (2012).
Regulation of the stress response by
the gut microbiota: Implications for
psychoneuroendocrinology.
Psychoneuroendocrinology, 37(9), 1369–1378.

Diniz, Breno Satler; Machado-Vieira,
Rodrigo; Forlenza, Orestes Vicente
(2013)
Lithium and neuroprotection: translational
evidence and implications for the treatment of neuropsychiatric disorders.
Neuropsychiatric disease and treatment vol. 9
p. 493-500

Dvoráková M, Jezová D, Blazícek P,
Trebatická J, Skodácek I, Suba J, Iveta W,
Rohdewald P, Duracková Z. (2007)
Urinary catecholamines in children with
attention deficit hyperactivity disorder
(ADHD): modulation by a polyphenolic
extract from pine bark (pycnogenol).
Nutritional neuroscience 10:3-4 pg 151-7
(01 June 2007)

Dubuc, Bruno
The Brain from Top to Bottom
Institute of Neurosciences, Mental Health
and Addiction
Canadian Institutes of Health Research
Ottawa, ON, K1A 0W9
http://thebrain.mcgill.ca/avance.php
Accessed 31 August 2014

Dyall, S C; Michael-Titus, A T (2008)
Neurological benefits of omega-3 fatty acids.
Neuromolecular medicine vol. 10 (4) p.
219-35

Edenberg, Howard J (2007)
The genetics of alcohol metabolism: role
of alcohol dehydrogenase and aldehyde
dehydrogenase variants.
*Alcohol research & health : the journal of the
National Institute on Alcohol Abuse and
Alcoholism* vol. 30 (1) p. 5-13

Eisenhofer, Graeme; Kopin, Irwin J.;
Goldstein, David S. (2004)

Catecholamine Metabolism: A
Contemporary View with Implications
for Physiology and Medicine
Pharmacol. Rev. vol. 56 (3) p. 331-349

Elan D. Louis, Pam Factor-Litvak, Marina
Gerbin, Wendy Jiang, and Wei Zheng,
"Blood Harmane Concentrations in 497
Individuals Relative to Coffee, Cigarettes,
and Food Consumption on the Morning
of Testing,"
Journal of Toxicology, vol. 2011.
doi:10.1155/2011/628151

Elsas, S-M; Rossi, D J; Raber, J; White, G;
Seeley, C-A et al. (2010)
Passiflora incarnata L. (Passionflower) extracts elicit GABA currents in hippocam-
pal neurons in vitro, and show anxiogenic
and anticonvulsant effects in vivo, varying
with extraction method.
*Phytomedicine : international journal of phy-
totherapy and phytopharmacology* vol. 17
(12) p. 940-9

Encyclopaedia Britannica
Alkaloid
*http://www.britannica.com/EBchecked/
topic/15672/alkaloid*
Accessed 10 February 2015

el-Yazigi, A; Martin, C R; Siqueira, E B
(1988)
Concentrations of chromium, cesium, and
tin in cerebrospinal fluid of patients with
brain neoplasms, leukemia or other non-
cerebral malignancies, and neurological
diseases.
Clinical chemistry vol. 34 (6) p. 1084-6

Environmental Protection Agency
Polychlorinated Biphenyls (PCBs)
Health Effects of PCBs
*http://www.epa.gov/epawaste/hazard/tsd/
pcbs/pubs/effects.htm*
Accessed 10 February 2015

Fediuk, Daryl J; Wang, Tao; Raizman, Joshua
E; Parkinson, Fiona E; Gu, Xiaochen
(2010)

Tissue deposition of the insect repellent DEET and the sunscreen oxybenzone from repeated topical skin applications in rats.
International journal of toxicology vol. 29 (6) p. 594-603

Fernstrom, John D (2000)
Can nutrient supplements modify brain function?
Am J Clin Nutr vol. 71 (6) p. 1669S-1673

Foster, J. A., & McVey Neufeld, K.-A. (2013).
Gut–brain axis: how the microbiome influences anxiety and depression.
Trends in Neurosciences, 36(5), 305-312.

Fowler, B A (1978)
General subcellular effects of lead, mercury, cadmium, and arsenic.
Environmental health perspectives vol. 22 p. 37-41

Freeman, Roy, MD.
TREATMENT OF AUTONOMIC NEUROPATHY. Treatment of autonomic dysfunction of the gastrointestinal tract (Part three).
Harvard Medical School, Boston MA
http://www.neuropathy.org/site/DocServer/ Treatment_of_Autonomic_Neuropathy_-_ Gastrointestinal_Sym.pdf retrieved 18 November 2014.

Gautam, Medhavi; Agrawal, Mukta; Gautam, Manaswi; Sharma, Praveen; Gautam, Anita Sharma et al. (2012)
Role of antioxidants in generalised anxiety disorder and depression.
Indian journal of psychiatry vol. 54 (3) p. 244-7

Gershon, Michael D (2013)
5-Hydroxytryptamine (serotonin) in the gastrointestinal tract.
Current opinion in endocrinology, diabetes, and obesity vol. 20 (1) p. 14-21

Goldstein, Randy J. MD
Hydrocarbons Toxicity
Medscape

http://emedicine.medscape.com/ article/1010734-overview
Accessed 16 February 2015

Grill, Marie F; Maganti, Rama K (2011)
Neurotoxic effects associated with antibiotic use: management considerations.
British journal of clinical pharmacology vol. 72 (3) p. 381-93

Grønli, Ole; Kvamme, Jan Magnus; Jorde, Rolf; Wynn, Rolf (2014)
Vitamin D deficiency is common in psychogeriatric patients, independent of diagnosis.
BMC psychiatry vol. 14 p. 134

Hahn, M K; Blakely, R D (2002)
Monoamine transporter gene structure and polymorphisms in relation to psychiatric and other complex disorders
Macmillan Publishers Limited vol. 2 (4) p. 217-235

Hashida, H; Honda, T; Morimoto, H; Aibara, Y (2001)A case of chronic bromvalerylurea intoxication due to habitual use of commercially available nonsteroidal anti-inflammatory drugs presenting an indefinite hyperchloremia.
Nihon Ronen Igakkai zasshi. Japanese journal of geriatrics vol. 38 (5) p. 700-3

Heijtz, Rochellys Diaz; Wang, Shugui; Anuar, Farhana; Qian, Yu; Bjorkholm, Britta et al. (2011)
Normal gut microbiota modulates brain development and behavior
PNAS vol. 108 (7) p. 3047-3052

Hyland, Keith (2007)
Inherited Disorders Affecting Dopamine and Serotonin: Critical Neurotransmitters Derived from Aromatic Amino Acids
J. Nutr. vol. 137 (6) p. 1568S-1572

Huang, Charles Lung-Cheng (2010)
The role of serotonin and possible interaction of serotonin-related genes with alcohol dehydrogenase and aldehyde dehydrogenase genes in alcohol dependence-a review.

American journal of translational research vol. 2 (2) p. 190-9

Hunt, Robert, MD (2006)
Functional Roles of Norepinephrine and Dopamine in ADHD: Dopamine in ADHD
Medscape Psychiatry. 2006;11(1)
Accessed 02 Dec 2014 *http://www.medscape.org/viewarticle/523887*

Hyman, Steven E. (2005)
Primer - Neurotransmitters
Current Biology Vol 15 No 5 R155

INCHEM
International Programme on Chemical Safety
http://www.inchem.org/
Accessed February 2015

Jacobus, Joanna; Tapert, Susan F (2013)
Neurotoxic effects of alcohol in adolescence.
Annual review of clinical psychology vol. 9 p. 703-21

Johansen, Espen Borgå; Knoff, Monica; Fonnum, Frode; Lausund, Per Leines; Walaas, S Ivar et al. (2011)
Postnatal exposure to PCB 153 and PCB 180, but not to PCB 52, produces changes in activity level and stimulus control in outbred male Wistar Kyoto rats.
Behavioral and brain functions : BBF vol. 7 p.

Kaidanovich-Beilin, Oksana; Cha, Danielle S; McIntyre, Roger S (2012)
Crosstalk between metabolic and neuropsychiatric disorders.
F1000 biology reports vol. 4 p. 14

Karama, S; Ducharme, S; Corley, J; Chouinard-Decorte, F; Starr, J M et al. (2015)
Cigarette smoking and thinning of the brain/'s cortex
Macmillan Publishers Limited

Katz, Kenneth D. MD, FAAEM, ABMT
Organophosphate Toxicity
Medscape

http://emedicine.medscape.com/article/167726-overview
Accessed 16 February 2015

Kidd, P.M. PhD. (2005) Neurodegeneration from Mitochondrial Insufficiency: Nutrients, Stem Cells, Growth Factors, and Prospects for Brain Rebuilding Using Integrative Management.
Alternative Medicine Review vol. 10 (4) p. 268-293.

Lakhan, Shaheen E. and Viera, Karen F.
Nutritional therapies for mental disorders.
Nutrition Journal 2008, 7:2
doi:10.1186/1475-2891-7-2

Lee, K.E., Langer, S.K., Barber, L.B., Writer, J.H., Ferrey, M.L., Schoenfuss, H.L., Furlong, E.T., William T. Foreman, Gray, J.L., ReVello, R.C., Martinovic, D., Woodruff, O.P., Keefe, S.H., Brown, G.K., Taylor, H.E., Ferrer, I., and Thurman, E.M., (2011)
Endocrine active chemicals, pharmaceuticals, and other chemicals of concern in surface water, wastewater-treatment plant effluent, and bed sediment, and biological characteristics in selected streams, Minnesota—design, methods, and data.
2009: U.S. Geological Survey Data Series 575, 54 p., with appendixes.

Lee, Wing-Hin; Loo, Ching-Yee; Bebawy, Mary; Luk, Frederick; Mason, Rebecca S et al. (2013)
Curcumin and its derivatives: their application in neuropharmacology and neuroscience in the 21st century.
Current neuropharmacology vol. 11 (4) p. 338-78

Lee, Yeonju; Jung, Jae-Chul; Jang, Soyong; Kim, Jieun; Ali, Zulfiqar et al. (2013)
Anti-Inflammatory and Neuroprotective Effects of Constituents Isolated from Rhodiola rosea.
Evidence-based complementary and alternative medicine : eCAM vol. 2013 p. 514049

Li, Hong; Zhou, Dinglun; Zhang, Qin; Feng, Chengyong; Zheng, Wei et al. (2013) Vanadium exposure-induced neurobehavioral alterations among Chinese workers. *NeuroToxicology* vol. 36 p. 49-54

Lin, Zhicheng; Canales, Juan J; Björgvinsson, Thröstur; Thomsen, Morgane; Qu, Hong et al. (2011) Monoamine transporters: vulnerable and vital doorkeepers. *Progress in molecular biology and translational science* vol. 98 p. 1-46

Linus pauling Micronutrient Information Center Oregon State University *http://lpi.oregonstate.edu/infocenter/* Accessed November and December 2014

Logan, Alan C; Jacka, Felice N (2014) Nutritional psychiatry research: an emerging discipline and its intersection with global urbanization, environmental challenges and the evolutionary mismatch. *Journal of physiological anthropology* vol. 33 p. 22

Lopetuso, Loris R; Scaldaferri, Franco; Petito, Valentina; Gasbarrini, Antonio (2013) Commensal Clostridia: leading players in the maintenance of gut homeostasis. *Gut pathogens* vol. 5 (1) p. 23

Lucchini,Roberto; Albini, Elisa. (2000) Mechanism of neurobehavioral alteration. *Toxicology letters* vol. 112-113 p. 35 - 9

Luissint, Anny-Claude; Artus, Cédric; Glacial, Fabienne; Ganeshamoorthy, Kayathiri; Couraud, Pierre-Olivier (2012) Tight junctions at the blood brain barrier: physiological architecture and disease-associated dysregulation. *Fluids and barriers of the CNS* vol. 9 (1) p. 23

Lyte, Mark (2013) Microbial Endocrinology in the Microbiome-Gut-Brain Axis: How Bacterial Production and Utilization of Neurochemicals Influence Behavior

PLoS Pathogens vol. 9 (11) p. 3

Manju A Kurian, Paul Gissen (2011) The monoamine neurotransmitter disorders: an expanding range of neurological syndromes. *Lancet neurology* vol. 10 (8) p. 721 - 33

Marchitti, Satori A.; Deitrich, Richard A.; Vasiliou, Vasilis (2007) Neurotoxicity and Metabolism of the Catecholamine-Derived 3,4-Dihydroxyphenylacetaldehyde and 3,4-Dihydroxyphenylglycolaldehyde: The Role of Aldehyde Dehydrogenase *Pharmacol. Rev.* vol. 59 (2) p. 125-150

Mayo Clinic Drugs and Supplements *http://www.mayoclinic.org/drugs-supplements/*

Medline Plus Encyclopedia (2014) The Mediterranean diet. *http://www.nlm.nih.gov/medlineplus/ency/patientinstructions/000110.htm* Accessed 14 November 2014

Millichap, J. Gordon; Yee, Michelle M. (2012) The Diet Factor in Attention-Deficit/ Hyperactivity Disorder *Pediatrics* vol. 129 (2) p. 330-337

Mirotti,L.; Castro, J; Costa-Pinto,F.A.; Russo, M. (2010) "Neural Pathways in Allergic Inflammation," *Journal of Allergy*, vol. 2010, Article ID 491928, doi:10.1155/2010/491928

Morey, Jeanine S.; Ryan, James C.; Bottein Dechraoui, Marie-Yasmine; Rezvani, Amir H.; Levin, Edward D. et al. (2008) Liver Genomic Responses to Ciguatoxin: Evidence for Activation of Phase I and Phase II Detoxification Pathways following an Acute Hypothermic Response in Mice *Toxicol. Sci.* vol. 103 (2) p. 298-310

Morgan, Edward T. (2001) Regulation of Cytochrome P450 by Inflammatory Mediators: Why and How?

Drug Metab. Dispos. vol. 29 (3) p. 207-212

Muntauu, Ania C. M.D. et al. (2002)
Tetrahydrobiopterin as an Alternative
Treatment for Mild Phenylketonuria
N Engl J Med 2002;
347:2122-2132December 26, 2002DOI:
10.1056/NEJMoa021654

Nabeshima, Toshitaka; Kim, Hyoung-Chun
(2013)
Involvement of genetic and environmental
factors in the onset of depression.
Experimental neurobiology vol. 22 (4) p.
235-43

National Institute on Drug Abuse.
Impacts of Drugs on Neurotransmission
*http://www.drugabuse.gov/news-
events/nida-notes/2007/10/
impacts-drugs-neurotransmission*
Accessed 17 February 2015

Nelson, Erika D; Monteggia, Lisa M (2011)
Epigenetics in the mature mammalian
brain: effects on behavior and synaptic
transmission.
Neurobiology of learning and memory vol. 96
(1) p. 53-60

Nezami, Behtash Ghazi; Srinivasan, Shanthi
(2010)
Enteric nervous system in the small intestine: pathophysiology and clinical
implications.
Current gastroenterology reports vol. 12 (5) p.
358-65

Benzo[a]pyrene-induced neurobehavioral
function and neurotransmitter alterations
in coke oven workers.
Niu, Qiao; Zhang, Hongmei; Li, Xin; Li,
Meiqin (2010)
Occupational and environmental medicine vol.
67 (7) p. 444-8

Numakawa, Tadahiro; Richards, Misty;
Nakajima, Shingo; Adachi, Naoki; Furuta,
Miyako et al. (2014)
The role of brain-derived neurotrophic
factor in comorbid depression: possible

linkage with steroid hormones, cytokines,
and nutrition.
Frontiers in psychiatry vol. 5 p. 136

Obayashi, Patsy, MS, RD, CDE. (2006)
Healthy Nutrition, Healthy Liver
Department of Clinical Nutrition
Stanford Hospital and Clinics

Olson, Christopher R; Mello, Claudio V
(2010)
Significance of vitamin A to brain function,
behavior and learning.
Molecular nutrition & food research vol. 54
(4) p. 489-95

OMIM – Online Mendelian Inheritance in
Man
http://omim.org/
Accessed 10 December 2014

Occupational Safety and Health
Administration (OSHA)
United States Department of Labor
Toluene Standards
*https://www.osha.gov/SLTC/toluene/stan-
dards.html*
Accessed 23 January 2015

Patrick, Rhonda P.; Ames, Bruce N. (2015)
Vitamin D and the omega-3 fatty acids control serotonin synthesis and action, part
2: relevance for ADHD, bipolar, schizophrenia, and impulsive behavior
FASEB J p. fj.14-268342-

Pesticide Action Network of North America
PAN Pesticide Database
http://www.pesticideinfo.org/
Accessed February 2015

Pelusser, Lidy M. et al. (2011)
Eff ects of a restricted elimination diet on
the behaviour of children with atten-
tion-defi cit hyperactivity disorder
(INCA study): a randomised controlled trial
The Lancet,Vol 377 February 5, 2011

Purvis, Karen, et al (2006)
An Experimental Evaluation of Targeted
Amino Acid Therapy with At-Risk
Children. Poster

Scripps Center for Integrative Medicine 2006 Conference. La Jolla, CA.

Putschögl, Franziska Maria; Gaum, Petra Maria; Schettgen, Thomas; Kraus, Thomas; Gube, Monika et al. (2015) Effects of occupational exposure to polychlorinated biphenyls on urinary metabolites of neurotransmitters: A cross-sectional and longitudinal perspective
International Journal of Hygiene and Environmental Health vol. 218 (5) p. 452-460

Rahman, M Khalilur; Choudhary, M Iqbal; Arif, M; Morshed, M Monzur (2014) Dopamine- -Hydroxylase Activity and Levels of Its Cofactors and Other Biochemical Parameters in the Serum of Arsenicosis Patients of Bangladesh.
International journal of biomedical science : IJBS vol. 10 (1) p. 52-60

Rao, T S Sathyanarayana; Asha, M R; Ramesh, B N; Rao, K S Jagannatha (2008) Understanding nutrition, depression and mental illnesses.
Indian journal of psychiatry vol. 50 (2) p. 77-82

Ross, Brian M; Seguin, Jennifer; Sieswerda, Lee E (2007) Omega-3 fatty acids as treatments for mental illness: which disorder and which fatty acid?
Lipids in health and disease vol. 6 p. 21

Rutten, Bart P F; Mill, Jonathan (2009) Epigenetic mediation of environmental influences in major psychotic disorders.
Schizophrenia bulletin vol. 35 (6) p. 1045-56

Sauve, Anthony A. (2008) NAD+ and Vitamin B3: From Metabolism to Therapies
J. Pharmacol. Exp. Ther. vol. 324 (3) p. 883-893

Scanlon, Richard, A. PhD Nitrosamines and Cancer The Linus Pauling Institute

http://lpi.oregonstate.edu/f-w00/nitrosamine.html
Accessed 16 February 2015

Semple, S (2004) Dermal exposure to chemicals in the workplace: just how important is skin absorption?
Occup. Environ. Med. vol. 61 (4) p. 376-382

Singh, Ranvir; White, Mark A. (2006) Structure of a glutathione conjugate bound to the active site of aldose reductase.
Proteins vol. 64 (1) p. 101 - 10

Shao, Andrew; Hathcock, John N (2008) Risk assessment for the amino acids taurine, L-glutamine and L-arginine.
Regulatory toxicology and pharmacology : RTP vol. 50 (3) p. 376-99

Shepherd, Janet E. (2001) Effects of Estrogen on Cognition, Mood, and Degenerative Brain Diseases.
J Am Pharm Assoc. 2001;41(2)

Shih, J C; Chen, K; Ridd, M J (1999) Monoamine oxidase: from genes to behavior.
Annual review of neuroscience vol. 22 p. 197-217

Stevens, Laura J; Kuczek, Thomas; Burgess, John R; Stochelski, Mateusz A; Arnold, L Eugene et al. (2013) Mechanisms of behavioral, atopic, and other reactions to artificial food colors in children
Nutrition Reviews vol. 71 (5) p. 268-281

Szegedi, A; Kohnen, R; Dienel, A; Kieser, M (2005) Acute treatment of moderate to severe depression with hypericum extract WS 5570 (St John's wort): randomised controlled double blind non-inferiority trial versus paroxetine.
BMJ (Clinical research ed.) vol. 330 (7490) p. 503

Thompson, R.F. (2000). The Brain: A Neuroscience Primer. New York: Worth Publishers.

Triebig, G; Hallermann, J (2001)
Survey of solvent related chronic enceph-
alopathy as an occupational disease in
European countries
Occup. Environ. Med. vol. 58 (9) p. 575-581

Twigt, Bas A; Houweling, Bernard M; Vriens,
Menno R; Regeer, Eline J; Kupka, Ralph
W et al. (2013)
Hypercalcemia in patients with bipolar dis-
order treated with lithium: a cross-sec-
tional study.
International Journal of Bipolar Disorders vol.
1 (1) p. 18

University of Utah
Learn.Genetics Genetic Science Learning
Center
Epigenetics and Inheritance
*http://learn.genetics.utah.edu/content/
epigenetics/inheritance/*
Accessed 22 January 2015

van Donkelaar, Eva L; Vaessen, Koen R D;
Pawluski, Jodi L; Sierksma, Annerieke S;
Blokland, Arjan et al. (2014)
Long-term corticosterone exposure decreas-
es insulin sensitivity and induces depres-
sive-like behaviour in the C57BL/6NCrl
mouse.
PloS one vol. 9 (10) p. e106960

Virgolini, Miriam B.; Chen, Kevin; Weston,
Doug D.; Bauter, Mark R.; Cory-Slechta,
Deborah A. (2005)
Interactions of Chronic Lead Exposure
and Intermittent Stress: Consequences
for Brain Catecholamine Systems and
Associated Behaviors and HPA Axis
Function
Toxicol. Sci. vol. 87 (2) p. 469-482

Washington Department of Fish & Wildlife
Razor Clams
DOMOIC ACID - A major concern to
washington state's shellfish lovers
*http://wdfw.wa.gov/fishing/shellfish/razor-
clams/domoic_acid.html*
Accessed 17 February 2015

WebMD

Natural Medicines Comprehensive Database
Professional Version. © Therapeutic
Research Faculty 2009.
www.webmd.com
Accessed December 2014 and January 2015.

Wharton, Whitney; Gleason, Carey E; Olson,
Sandra R M S; Carlsson, Cynthia M;
Asthana, Sanjay (2012)
Neurobiological Underpinnings of the
Estrogen - Mood Relationship.
Current psychiatry reviews vol. 8 (3) p.
247-256

Widy-Tyszkiewicz, Ewa; Piechal, Agnieszka;
Gajkowska, Barbara; miałek, Mieczysław
(2002)
Tellurium-induced cognitive deficits in rats
are related to neuropathological changes
in the central nervous system
Toxicology Letters vol. 131 (3) p. 203-214

Wright, Robert O.; Baccarelli, Andrea (2007)
Metals and Neurotoxicology
J. Nutr. vol. 137 (12) p. 2809-2813

Yuan, Hong; He, Shuchang; He, Mingwei;
Niu, Qiao; Wang, Lei et al. (2006)
A comprehensive study on neurobehav-
ior, neurotransmitters and lymphocyte
subsets alteration of Chinese manganese
welding workers.
Life sciences vol. 78 (12) p. 1324-8

Zhang, H., Yan, Y., Shi, R., Lin, Z., Wang, M.,
& Lin, L. (2008).
Correlation of gut hormones with irritable
bowel syndrome.
Digestion, 78(2-3), 72–6.
doi:10.1159/000165352

Zhang, Xiang; Ho, Shuk-Mei (2011)
Epigenetics meets endocrinology
J. Mol. Endocrinol. vol. 46 (1) p. R11-32

Zheng, Ping (2009)
Neuroactive steroid regulation of neurotransmitter release in the CNS: action,
mechanism and possible significance.
Progress in neurobiology vol. 89 (2) p. 134-52

Zhou, Feng C; Balaraman, Yokesh; Teng, MingXiang; Liu, Yunlong; Singh, Rabindra P et al. (2011)
Alcohol alters DNA methylation patterns and inhibits neural stem cell differentiation.
Alcoholism, clinical and experimental research vol. 35 (4) p. 735-46

Zucchi, R; Chiellini, G; Scanlan, T S; Grandy, D K (2006)
Trace amine-associated receptors and their ligands.
British journal of pharmacology vol. 149 (8) p. 967-78